A Clinician's Guide to Assessing Mental Health Emergencies:

A Field Manual For Assessing Risk

Written by Brooks Baer, M.A., L. C. P. C.
Edited by Blake Passmore, M. Ed., L. C. P. C.

ISBN: 978-0-9889549-1-5

Library of Congress Control Number: 2013932940

Published In The United States Of America
Printed in Canada

**To purchase additional copies
or inquire regarding training workshops**

visit: www.psychrisk.com

Published and Distributed by:

PsychRisk, LLC
175 Hutton Ranch Rd., Ste. 103
Kalispell, MT 59901
www.psychrisk.com
1 (800) 407-1549
email: info@psychrisk.com

Foreword by Dr. Richard Briles

This book addresses a large problem facing many practicing clinicians: the organized assessment and practical disposition of the mental health crisis patient. The book will be useful to many types of clinicians including psychiatrists, emergency physicians, primary care physicians, psychologists, social workers, therapists and mental health professionals. I am an Emergency Physician and working with mental health patients is regular part of my job. Like any clinician, I am trained to seek a variety of data sources to make clinical decisions. I prefer to rely on objective data obtained from history, physical examination, radiological and laboratory data, etc. Hopefully all this information tidies up into a neat little package called a diagnosis, which then leads to a treatment plan and most importantly a patient disposition. Unfortunately, for most clinicians including myself, this process tends to break down in the evaluation of the mental health crisis patient. The history is frequently vague or conflicting. Too often it comes down to believing either 'what he said or she said'. Physical exam is usually not helpful and frequently the patient is not cooperative. Ancillary data, with the exception or drug and alcohol testing, rarely sheds light on the issue. Frequently, we become frustrated by the lack of concrete data and conflicting information presented that prevents us from using reliable methods to come to clinical decisions. At that point any hope of coming to a neat little diagnosis and firm disposition plan is usually out the window so we come to conclusions like "He's really crazy", "He's just really drunk or stoned" or "He seems really depressed". We then sometimes throw up our hands and are forced to go with our "gut feeling", or worse yet, "fly by the seat of our pants on this one".

Brooks Baer has put together a manual, or more specifically a method, for clinicians to efficiently navigate through the chaos involved in mental health crisis assessment. What the manual does is teach us how to efficiently make rational decisions out of frequently irrational situations. What I found unique about the manual is it is written from the perspective of the health provider. It addresses equally the problems clinicians face in dealing with mental health crisis patients as well as providing solid clinical advice on how to manage them. The basic tenant in the book is that two essential criteria must be met prior to every patient disposition: the safety of the patient and/or society as well minimizing liability of the health care practitioner.

The book is written is such a way that it will be useful to a wide variety of practitioners. It is a quick read so I recommend you initially read it cover to cover. It should take only a few hours, a day or two at most. It is well organized, devoid of esoterica, so it works well as quick go to pocket reference. You could consider it a "Mental Health Crisis Evaluation for Dummies" for physicians like me whose practice involves relatively small numbers of these patients but a large percentage of total angst and frustration. It is also thorough enough to be used as a core reference for psychiatrists, MHP's, and crisis therapists who work with these patients on a regular basis.

As a practicing MHP, Brooks has evaluated thousands of these patients in places like ER's, mental health clinics and correctional facilities. His method for evaluation of mental health crisis patients is a tried and true technique honed over years of practice. As an educator, he now travels the country giving weekly seminars on this topic and has spent countless hours researching the subject matter. The basic tenants espoused in the book are backed by a comprehensive volume of research. I feel this book has filled a large gap in my clinical practice and has been one of the most practical references I have ever used. If your practice also involves the evaluation of the mental health crisis patient I'm sure you will come to the same conclusion.

Richard W. Briles, MD

The Writer And Editor

Brooks Baer, M. A., L.C.P.C.

Brooks has over 20 years of experience. He is a Risk Assessment Specialist and routinely performs psychiatric evaluations in a variety of contexts (e.g. ER, psychiatric hospital, jail). Brooks frequently offers expert testimony in court commitment proceedings, and he provides mobile crisis response for the Western Montana Mental Health Center.

In addition, Brooks has a busy private practice, where he keeps in touch with the situations most counselors face in their offices. He has also taught for the University of Great Falls, MT. In his many seminars, Brooks uses humor and peer based discussion groups to engage listeners and to facilitate maximum retention.

Brooks has a passion for research and writing. He can frequently be seen in airports typing manuscripts for his next presentation or book as he travels across the country from his home in Northwest Montana to present training workshops on numerous topics related to mental health assessment.

Blake Passmore, M. Ed., L. C. P. C.

Blake has over 22 years of experience in public mental health. He is a Risk Assessment Specialist and routinely performs psychiatric evaluations in a variety of contexts (e.g. ER, psychiatric hospital, jail). Blake provides mobile crisis response for the Western Montana Mental Health Center.

As part of his responsibilities, Blake regularly testifies as a Certified Professional Person for involuntary commitment hearings for individuals who meet commitment criteria set by state statutes.

Blake also has extensive background in public mental health services as a therapist and clinical supervisor in a rural mental health center as well as a large mental health center serving in a county with a population of nearly 100,000. Blake has also practiced as a private mental health clinician and as a pastoral counselor.

In addition to his professional career, Blake also has a variety of experience in the business field. His greatest business success has been starting a small publishing company. He also is a frequent contributor for an on-line recreation community and has released a guidebook series on climbing in Glacier National Park.

Purpose

The purpose of this workbook is three-fold. First, to increase your ability to recognize the underlying conditions that increase suicide risk. Second, to help you make an informed decision regarding your patient's ability to cope with traumatic stressors. Third, to formulate an appropriate disposition for that patient.

Arriving at the correct dispositions requires us to make a clinical decision based on the patient's presentation, possible mental illnesses, coping mechanisms and current circumstances in life. Making this informed clinical decision is the best we can do. Risk assessment is never a sure thing and in many ways is an unreasonable task - but it is a task that needs to be performed. My goal is to assist you in this task.

Acknowledgement

I have been fortunate to work with dozens of psychiatrists and Emergency Department physicians over the past 15 years. I have learned something from them all. I would like to mention the few who had the most influence on me but I am reluctant to associate their names with all of the concepts in this interview guide. I do not want anyone to be held accountable for my thoughts and opinions.

Table Of Contents

Introduction

Part One: The Clinical Interview

Clinical Disorders

Part Two: Specific Risk Inquiry

Part Three: Disposition

Appendix

Introduction

After teaching hundreds of seminars to thousands of clinicians I am occasionally confronted after a seminar with a statement such as this: *"You still haven't told us who is safe and who isn't. I came here so I could learn who will kill themselves and who won't!"* I respond to this statement with the simple fact that there is no secret formula for risk assessment. There is no way to know for sure who is safe and who isn't. I can't give you "10 Handy Rules" for suicide assessment. That is not the purpose of this workbook. The purpose of this workbook is to bring structure to the complex task of risk assessment.

While any clinician is welcome to utilize this workbook - it is written for the risk assessment professional who is asked on a day-to-day basis to evaluate patients in high risk settings (such as Emergency Departments and Community Crisis Centers). This workbook is intended to provide a framework that depicts a consistent means of evaluating patients who appear to be at risk for violence towards self or others.

Perhaps an analogy will help set the framework for conducting risk interviews. The flu kills thousands of people a year in the United States. This statement is both true and false. People with the flu do die every year; worldwide hundreds of thousands a year die. But did the flu kill them? The flu does not necessarily kill by its self; the flu kills medically compromised individuals. They were in a weakened condition and the flu overwhelmed their immune system. To say that they died from the flu is not entirely accurate.

Suicide is similar. People who are emotionally compromised encounter the same stressors that millions of other people successfully overcome. People lose jobs, get sick, have loved ones die, and relationships end. These heartbreaking events occur daily around the world - but for some, these events prove to be more than they can cope with. They were already in an emotionally-weakened condition and their "emotional immune system" became overwhelmed. This may be the result of a clinical condition such as depression or post-traumatic stress disorder, or it may be a personality disorder. It is our job to understand and recognize these compromising disorders and identify those individuals who are currently encountering a stressor that is more overwhelming than they can manage.

In addition, we need to understand the nature of the "emotional immune system". What is it that allows most people to successfully cope with traumatic changes in life? What are some people missing? The short answer is this. Relationships appear to be the key to a robust emotional immune system. This is not to imply that one must be in a relationship in order to be emotionally healthy but it is true that relationships boost emotional immunity. A much longer answer is previous relationships - or primarily, attachment relationships. The value of current relationships is obvious provided the individuals are supportive of each other. The value of attachment relationships may not be so obvious on the surface but there is a great deal of research that supports the idea that infant attachment provides a significant foundation for emotional resilience. In the absence of attachment, many people find themselves without the ability to cope with some of the more significant changes of life.

Research reveals that most suicide is precipitated by relationship losses. It is my belief that infant attachments provide a cushion that allows people to rebound from current relationship losses. People can draw relational currency from these internal attachments that sustain them until they repair or replace current relationships. Most of our suicide assessments will involve individuals with some degree of current relationship loss. It should be noted that relationships do not play a major role in psychotic suicides.

What Is Risk Assessment?

It is extremely difficult to quantify "risk". It is not difficult to recognize the "quality" of risk. We know when it is present - we simply struggle to assign a number or value to it. In the management of psychiatric risk we rarely get objective data to analyze. We are primarily working with patient reports and our subjective interpretation of our patient. At best a reliable collateral source illuminates our patient for us. Occasionally the collateral source is as impaired as the patient. What then do we rely upon for making these life or death decisions?

Should we rely on our intuition when determining risk? I always listen to my intuition when it tells me someone is at risk. I never listen to my intuition when it tells me to let someone go home. The only way someone goes home is if the case documentation supports an outpatient disposition. In the event of a suicide you need to be bringing more into court than your intuition - which was clearly in error.

A simple rule that has guided me in thousands of cases. I use the "man on the street test" also known as the "reasonable person test."

It important to note that in court, the "reasonable person" will always be presented as a perfect individual who always makes the right decision. Of course, this imaginary perfect person will be evaluated in the light of hindsight. You clearly do not have the benefit of hindsight; your decisions must be made in the darkness of potential deception and conflicting goals on the part of the various stakeholders in the situation. In addition you may be several cases deep in a busy Emergency Department with busy doctors, nurses and law enforcement officers all wanting you to clear their case first.

The Man On The Street Test

"What would the average person on the street think of this situation?" Some clinicians say to me: "Who cares what the average person thinks? We are the professionals."

While it is obviously true that we are the professionals, it is also true that professionals do not sit on juries - average people do. All of our decisions must make sense to the average person or we run the risk of a malpractice finding in the event of a bad outcome. Evaluate and document with juries in mind, not colleagues.

The Patient

You cannot assume that you and the patient share a common goal. Occasionally you will, but more often your goals will be competing. A psychiatrist friend often said to me: "Remember, Brooks - these are adversarial interviews." He didn't mean that we should act like adversaries; he simply wanted to remind me to approach the situation with suspicion and not assume the patient was being truthful.

Collateral Source Or Sources

In most cases there is a husband, wife, family member or friend who has been involved in this unfolding drama for days. They have critical information that you must consider - even if you don't accept it as fact. We need to keep in mind that they may have an agenda of their own. It may be as simple as getting rid of their needy friend or family member so they can go on a trip or it may be related to custody disputes - the possibilities for manipulation are endless.

The Emergency Room Physician

Their perspective should primarily be colored by patient safety. The safest move for the physician is to hospitalize the patient, there is no risk involved in this disposition. Their desire for safety must be balanced by the admitting psychiatrist who knows how impossible it is to admit every patient who threatens to kill themselves. This would quickly overwhelm the mental health care system and no one would get help.

Law Enforcement

They too are motivated by patient safety but typically they are also motivated by the desire to see the situation resolved - they don't want to respond to the same situation again and again. This is reasonable but not always attainable.

Your Primary Goal:

Safety for the patient and safety for the community.

No other goal has any standing with you.

When you are feeling particularly pressured by other stakeholders ask yourself, "What would you do in their absence?"

If it was just you and the patient - what would you do?

As much as possible make every effort to reduce crisis situations down to the core elements.

What establishes risk and what is the least restrictive way to insure the safety of the patient and community?

You determine if the patient made statements or engaged in actions that substantiates risk.

You then formulate a legal and clinically sound plan to mitigate that risk.

A Three-Fold Perspective Of Assessment

I evaluate patients from three different perspectives: the patient, the situation, and the potential trajectory. Imagine a scenario such as this: a husband returns home drunk - with half of his paycheck gone. His wife reminds him that she told him she would leave him if this happened again. As she begins to pack her things he gets a gun and tells her to simply shoot him. He says: "I love you so much. If you leave me it will kill me. Just shoot me and get it done." He then holds the gun to his head, and tries to get her to take it. He puts it to his chest and says, "Just pull the trigger. Leaving me will kill me anyway." Eventually she gives in and tells him she will stay. He puts the gun down and goes into the kitchen - she calls 911. The police then transport the patient to the ER and you are expected to make sense of the situation.

By the time you evaluate the patient he is sober. He tells you that he had no intention of killing himself; he states that the gun was not even loaded. He says, "I just needed her to know how much she means to me." After some discussion you come to believe him - this was simply a drunk, manipulative incident and there appears to be no ongoing acute risk. He further states reasons to live. He is convincing and sincere. Your clinical impression is that he had no intention of taking his life and is not likely to ever take his life. If you are making a purely clinical decision you would discharge this patient. Risk management, however, is not always a purely clinical matter.

You must consider the elements of the situation: conflict, alcohol, a weapon, threats of suicide, extremely poor judgment, and law enforcement. Should all of these elements be dismissed because he is repentant? There is no way to know what the situation will be like when the patient returns home from the ER. He may be emboldened by his ability to convince both law enforcement and mental health professionals to see his point of view. He may be angry and feel betrayed that she called 911 and embarrassed him in the community. He may start drinking again and the situation may repeat with more intensity. She may be frustrated that no one takes her seriously. She may have been packing her things while he was at the ER. She may have been drinking.

This is a situation that the patient has created by their words and actions. Someone must bear the consequences of those words and actions - it will be you, or the patient. The patient will want you to bear the risk and take responsibility by letting them go home. Obviously this is not wise.

I recall a nurse early one morning who felt I was over reacting to a situation. He said: "There is a one-in-five-hundred chance that the person will kill themselves." I agreed with him and in those years I was managing over 500 cases a year - I told him that I didn't think the hospital would want to get sued once or twice a year because I failed to make people take responsibility for their actions.

If you are a career crisis manager then the odds are against you and the numbers will eventually catch up. Do everything you can to limit bad outcomes. If you are not a career crisis manager it is even more important to follow fairly rigid guidelines as you may miss crucial elements in the midst of complex and occasionally chaotic situations.

I. The Patient

We first evaluate the patient to determine if there is a mental illness present. This includes both clinical disorders and personality disorders. If we feel there is a mental illness present we then have to determine if the symptoms of that mental illness have created imminent risk. Personality disordered risk is more difficult to manage and we will discuss that later.

II. The Situation

Not all mental health emergencies have an "index event" - some simply arise out of a chronic condition that has reached a critical point. In most cases we do have an index event and you need to interview all collateral sources who were present during the event. Clearly you will have to determine who may or may not be making a good faith statement. It is always a mistake to believe that the patient is telling the truth. You don't have to treat them like they are lying but you must keep in mind that mental health emergencies are generally hostile situations where people have competing and conflicting agendas.

Your agenda is simple: you do the least intrusive thing that makes the situation safe for the patient and others. This will rarely make everyone happy. As you know, your job is not to make people happy; it is to diminish risk. This will require a calm, confident approach.

III. The Potential Trajectory

We need to have a bit of foresight and project where this situation is likely to go in the very near future. In addition to trajectory we are concerned with inertia, or: how much momentum does this situation have?

It is possible to deflect some of that momentum such as requiring a patient to spend the night with a friend or other family member rather than return home to a potentially hostile and agitated spouse? Keep in mind that while you may ask a patient to stay with other family members or friends you have no way of ensuring compliance with such a request.

It is your job to anticipate the worst case scenario and put a plan in place that diminishes risk factors associated with that scenario. This defensive way of practicing mental health may be foreign to some of you as it requires the assumption of the worst in everyone. This is the role of the risk manager.

> Never assume risk for another person: if they created a potentially dangerous and hostile situation then the responsibility must fall appropriately on them.

Index Event:

The event or series of events leading to the need for medical presentation.

Develop A Long Term Perspective On Crisis Management

Approach crisis management from an extremely defensive legal position.

Some clinicians suggest that we ignore legal concerns and focus on good patient care.

I am of the opinion that close attention to legal issues leads to good patient care. If this is your career, establish a long-term perspective that will guide you through the thousands of interviews you will conduct.

Medical Care Prior To Assessment

If the patient is to be seen at the medical facility a medical evaluation prior to your arrival is critical. Prior to the mental health assessment it is necessary to rule out any co-occurring medical issues that could possibly be the cause or even contributing factor for the current mental health condition that the patient is experiencing.

I feel that a brief physical examination by a physician as well as blood work and urinary analysis is crucial for accurate patient disposition. Without this important piece of information the clinician is beginning an assessment with only half of the picture. Many times medical evaluation identifies presence of a medical condition which when resolved has alleviated the patient's mental health concerns. For example, thyroid problems can contribute to individuals having anxiety - like symptoms. Brain tumors can contribute to thought disorders. Blood work can identify if a patient has a toxic level of lithium.

If a voluntary or involuntary admission are necessary the admitting psychiatric facility will want to have complete test results from the patient's blood as well as urinary analysis. They will also need physician notes as well as any collateral information gathered while the patient has been in the medical facility.

Although each inpatient facility is unique here are the recommended tests for ruling out physiological issues prior to inpatient admission.

Also included is basic security protocol for all mental health assessments.

Recommended Medical Screening

- Alcohol Level
- CBC with Diff
- CMP (Chem-12 or Comprehensive Medical Panel)
- Drugs of Abuse Screen, Urine
- SED Rate
- Triglycerides Level
- TSH
- Urinalysis

Staying Safe During Interviews:

Personal safety is paramount during the interview process.

Consider the following tips to remain safe.

- Know as much as you can about the patient prior to beginning the interview.
- Talk to the person who brought the patient for the risk assessment. It may be law enforcement, EMT or family members.
- Do not close the door and stand or sit closest to the open door.
- Maintain a safe personal distance from the patient.
- Be situationally aware of the surroundings.
- Look for items that could be used as weapons and ask for their removal.
- Ask law enforcement or security to either stand outside of the room or inside of the room as an added layer of safety.
- Maintain a relaxed posture with an open stance.
- Do not carry weapons, such as clipboards and pens, into the interview room.
- Avoid prolonged direct eye contact. Some patients interpret this behavior as challenging them.
- Tell the patient that you expect them to stay calm.
- Set clear boundaries. Tell the patient that threats of violence or acts of violence are unacceptable.
- If the patient becomes aggressive postpone the risk assessment until he or she can assessed without danger.
- Consider managing this patient's aggressive behaviors with medications or restraints as needed.

Recommended Security Protocol

- Request security for standby assist
- Separate patient from all belongings
- Undress patient
- Search patient for contraband
- Place in scrubs or gown

Managing Multiple Cases

I believe the key to managing multiple cases is to ignore everything but the case in front of you. I will conduct a quick triage to determine the order I am going to put the cases in but I will not work on two cases at the same time. As a rule I will address the most violent and chaotic cases first. I never even pick up the next chart until I have completely documented the case I am on.

I have had partners who like to run the cases in a sort of "rough draft" format. They conduct interviews and made dispositions without doing final documentation until all of the cases were done, this worked well for them. You need to find a style that works for you. If I work in a rough draft format I know that I will not do a good job of documenting the case later. I need to do it as I go. Others feel the pressure to pick up the next case and therefore won't do a good job of documentation if they do the cases one at a time. Find your style and rhythm and don't allow others to take you from it.

Documentation is what insures that I haven't missed a step in the assessment process. This is especially true when I am fatigued and buried in cases. In the event of a bad outcome no one is going to give you a break because you are working on 3 hours of sleep and 5 cases deep in crisis. In court, every case will be viewed as if it occurred in the midst of a beautiful sunshiny day in which you had nothing to do but devote hours to that particular situation. As situations become more chaotic I slow down - this helps me avoid mistakes.

Seven Cases On The Board

A colleague was called to the emergency department at 0130 for a mental health assessment. After arriving and completing the case disposition there were an additional 6 cases to be seen. Prior to the development of medical software cases were written on a dry erase board. Mental health assessment was designated for six more cases. There were no other medical cases.

The colleague reviewed each case and then took each case one by one from initial contact to disposition.

After that run of risk assessments there were three voluntary admissions to inpatient treatment, one patient was placed on an involuntary hold (emergency detention) and the remaining three cases were discharged.

He consulted with the psychiatrist after each case and completed the seventh risk assessment at 0830.

The B-52

Occasionally, we see patients who are so belligerent that they refuse to cooperate after exhausting all of the techniques used for hostile interviews.

The patient continues to be verbally and/or physically aggressive. This may include vulgar speech, spitting, violence or threats of violence, or perhaps a homicidal or psychotic patient threatening to elope from the hospital when leaving is against medical advise. At this time we make a decision to place the patient on an involuntary hold.

We then consult with the emergency room physician and recommend that some type of restraint be placed on the patient to ensure their safety as well as the safety of others.

Generally, the physician orders an injection of Haldol, Ativan, and Benedryl. We generally, request security as well as other staff to present as a "show of force" to encourage the patient to cooperate with receiving the medication. Generally, this works and the injection is administered.

Hostile Interviews:

Occasionally you will have to conduct an interview with a hostile patient or perhaps a hostile collateral source. Here are some suggestions for responding to some of the most common themes you may encounter.

"You can't do this to me."

I never engage in a debate about what I can, or can't do. I generally say: "This is not about what I can do, it is about what I am required to do. When I determine that someone is putting themselves or others in danger because of a mental illness I am required to take protective action."

"I want to talk to my lawyer."

I get them a phone book and leave the room for 30 minutes. If I have notes to do I may write them or I simply go to the break room and eat cookies. I never engage in an argument over the legal issues. I have never had a lawyer get engaged in that type of situation. If one did show up at the ER I would simply hand them a copy of the civil statutes and go about my business. Most private lawyers want nothing to do with mental health law; this is reserved for the public defenders.

"I am going to lose my job/house/kids because of you."

I tell them that I am involved because of their actions and words. I remind them that I didn't go out and find them and create this situation. The situation is the result of their behavior.

"I don't have to talk to you."

I acknowledge that they don't have to talk to me but they do have to talk to someone. This generally requires that they be admitted to a psychiatric unit so they can be interviewed the next day by a psychiatrist. In most cases I will inform them of this and offer to come back to give them another chance to engage in a productive interview. I often make up an excuse to take a short break and return to the interview, most often the patient has calmed down unless they are in a manic episode or experiencing psychosis.

***"You are being rude to me." (or) "You are out to get me." (or)
"You don't like me."***

Many personality disorder patients have learned that they can get special and/or lenient treatment if they put people on the defensive.

Don't respond defensively. Simply inform them that a productive interview is not possible if they feel you are being unfair. You will have to admit them to a psychiatric unit where they can be seen by a psychiatrist tomorrow. I then tell them I have to respond to another situation but I will be back shortly to check on them before they go to the unit. When I return, most of them have abandoned their offensive strategy and are ready to engage in a productive interview. If not, I write the court petition that allows me to hospitalize them involuntarily.

The belligerent intoxicated patient.

Many times an Emergency Department physician will want you to evaluate a patient who "appears to be clinically sober." This means that on observation there are no signs of intoxication. In this case the liability rests with the physician who is qualified to make that decision. You will only want to insist on a lab result if you feel that the patient is not sober and you have a genuine fear that the patient will harm themselves upon discharge. Once a lab result is present you have to wait until the patient is legally sober before you can have a defendable outpatient discharge.

The Collateral Interview

It is not possible to overstate the importance of collateral interviews in high-risk situations. We need to assume that every patient is not engaged in a good faith interview - they are lying. This doesn't mean we treat them as an adversary but it does mean that we doubt everything they say. In addition, we also have to assume that the collateral source may in fact be adversarial as well - they lie too. In the end we will have to decide who we feel is making good faith statements. When the stories are conflicting you will clearly have to determine who you believe and state your opinion in your clinical record. Be sure to include all versions of the story in your record; this shows that you made an informed decision after considering all sides of the story or event.

As an example I may write: "This patient's spouse does not appear to be making a good faith statement. It appears that they are motivated by an effort to exert stability in a situation they feel is out of their control." I have interviewed many spouses who assure me that their partner is suffering from some form of mental disorder because they would "never leave me for another person" or they would "never drink or do drugs unless something was really wrong in their head."

Keep in mind that the collateral interview is your preview to the plaintiff's case should you be sued in the event of a bad outcome. This is your chance to address the issues raised without a judge and jury looking over your shoulder. I always take time with collateral sources to make them feel heard and understood. This does not mean that I always make them happy or do what they want me to.

I do always tell them that I understand their position and I wish I could do something to help them but I am bound by the limits of the law. I never want a potentially hostile party to feel that I simply didn't choose their side because I didn't like them. I want them to feel like I tried to help them but could not because of the limits of mental health laws. Even if I feel someone is completely out of line I rarely confront them. There is no gain in this and significant potential risk. We always need to keep in mind that the "narcissistic wound" heals slow and often requires the salve of retribution before people can move on. It is always my goal to leave people with the sense that I heard and respect them.

Family Relationships

Many times patients are so focused on wanting to leave that they desperately try any family member who will vouch for their safety. I recommend that you spend some time determining that there is actually a relationship with this family member.

In addition to determining their opinion about risk ask questions related to the date of last contact and their opinion of the quality of the relationship. I also feel that spouses, significant others, parents, adult children, and siblings are the preferred sources.

Long-time Relationships

Best friends or long-time friends can also be a good source of information. I believe it is important to establish the nature of their relationship and determine if this person is a reliable source of information. Gathering information from unreliable sources is ineffective at best.

Managing Personality Disorders

Many of our cases will involve personality disordered individuals, either as a patient or collateral source. It is important to remember that each of the four personalities within that cluster that has been defined as B personalities can share in the traits of the other three disorders. Rarely (if ever) will you meet a "pure" personality disorder, which is why they are grouped as clusters in the DSM-5® *. With this in mind we want to be on the alert for the defining characteristic of each personality in a crisis situation.

I. The Borderline As A Patient

The borderline as a patient will be very attention seeking, they will quickly try to enmesh you in their life either by vilification or idealization. They will love you or hate you depending on what you are doing. You will typically encounter the borderline patient in one of two scenarios. In one, they have threatened to kill themselves for manipulative reasons and someone called law enforcement. In this case the patient generally wants to make this situation go away - they will down play the threats and in some cases will simply deny making them. I prefer it when they admit to the threats as manipulative efforts. I feel this "good faith effort" to tell the truth allows me to form a more lenient disposition. When they insist that the collateral source is lying, it can be more difficult to discharge the patient as they do not appear to be engaged in a good faith interview.

The second scenario involves a borderline patient who wants admission to a psychiatric unit for secondary gain. Perhaps it is simply because they have run out of groceries or they have been kicked out of their friend's house. Maybe they need to punish someone who has not behaved in the manner they wish them to. Occasionally you can divert this admission by determining what their core goal is; sometimes you will be forced into compliance if the risk of the patient escalating appears too great.

Keep in mind that in a borderline patient's life everything is about them and for them. They have a very child-like perspective that results in an entirely egocentric world view. This patient will push you to pursue whatever course of action best suits them. Generally this will involve them either being the victim, savior, or the martyr.

---

* DSM-5® is a registered trademark of American Psychiatric Association

II. The Borderline As A Collateral Source

A collateral source who suffers from borderline personality disorder can be very challenging. They generally are attempting to use you as a weapon against someone else. Once you have determined that they are attempting to manipulate you it is time to move on as quickly as possible. It is not likely that you will ever win them over to your way of thinking and you may burn hours in the attempt.

III. The Narcissist As A Patient.

This patient will be shocked that you actually intend to hold them accountable for their actions. As a narcissist they will typically feel both entitled and misunderstood. They are likely to persistently retell their story in the belief that you will eventually see things their way. Make every effort to avoid a personal power struggle with this individual. If possible suggest that they call your supervisor, this may divert their energy long enough for you to resolve the current crisis by gaining more information from others or allowing them to expend their "righteous energy" by attempting to get you in trouble.

IV. The Narcissist As A Collateral Source

In a word this individual will be demanding. They will expect you to do what they tell you to and may become threatening if you don't. You will need to find a balance between making them feel heard while you maintain your course of action. You want them to get the idea that you would love to obey them but the law will not allow you to. I often suggest that they contact a Senator or House Representative to have the laws changed. This communicates to them that the decision is well above my pay grade and it appeals to their narcissistic sense of grandiosity as they imagine themselves arguing and winning their case to a legislative body.

V. The Antisocial As A Patient

All antisocial patients need to be viewed as dangerous exploitive predators. If we ever forget their true nature we may find ourselves in a very bad situation. They will do whatever they need to in order to accomplish their goal. Your task is to determine what their goal is and make an attempt to reconcile their goal with your goal. Do not get hostile and confrontational with antisocial individuals.

VI. The Antisocial As A Collateral Source

It is important to remember that antisocial personalities come in two varieties: blue collar and white collar. Both will want you to do what they tell you too, they will simply tell you in different ways. The blue collar antisocial can be threatening in overt and covert ways, but at their core they are physically aggressive and view violence as a reasonable strategy. White collar antisocial is generally very charismatic and articulate. They will persistently retell their position until you agree.

A Short Course On Malpractice

Malpractice falls within what is called tort law. A tort is an action "turned aside" - an action outside of the "standard of care." It is important to understand what is meant by the standard of care. Standards of care are community driven standards based on community resources. You can only determine what the appropriate standard of care is in your community by exploring the resources available to you, such as knowing how to get someone admitted to a psychiatric hospital or safe house.

An important step in avoiding malpractice is to understand what it consists of. A common misconception regarding malpractice is the thought that it is "outcome dependent". This is the belief that a bad outcome is always the result of malpractice. This may be true but is not necessarily true. Bad outcomes occur even when things are done correctly. The outcome is not on trial, the process of assessment is on trial. You are never in charge of the outcome, and always in charge of the assessment. Conduct a complete and well-documented assessment and you significantly diminish the odds that you will lose a malpractice law suit.

I believe that the most complete assessments are the result of a semi-structured interview that follows a prescribed path. One of the central components of malpractice is a failure to consider relevant and available information. The semi-structured interview helps you avoid this failure.

The Four D's Of Malpractice

Duty - *You had a duty to treat the patient.*

Deviation - *You deviated from the standard of care.*

Damage - *Damage occurred to the patient.*

Directly Attributable - *The damage can be directly attributed to your deviation.*

Conducting The Semi-Structured Interview

The semi-structured interview is the best format if you are conducting a defensive assessment.

As stated, I always conduct a defensive assessment. Assume the worst possible outcome and build the case to defend against it. I believe this interview, as opposed to an "ad hoc clinical" interview will be easier to defend as I have conducted a more systematic search for risk factors.

> **Part One:** This workbook follows an established order but you frequently do not perform the interview in this same sequence. You ultimately must explore each domain, but not necessarily in any particular order.

PART ONE: The Clinical Interview

Clinical Disorders

I.	Substance Abuse
II.	Mood Disorders
III.	Anxiety Disorders
IV.	Schizophrenia and Other Psychotic Disorders
V.	Schizoaffective Disorder
VI.	Delusional Disorders
VII.	Eating Disorders
VIII.	Insomnia
IX.	Personality Disorders

Medical Disorders
Psychosocial Stressors
Psychotic Violence Inquiry

> **Part Two:** Much of the information you gain here is simply an act of "due diligence". You are demonstrating that you have sought out relevant and available information so that you can make an informed decision. Some of the information will not be of tremendous clinical value; it may simply have legal value in the event you have to defend your disposition in the event of a bad outcome.

Part Two: Specific Risk Inquiry

> **Part Three:** This is where you formulate a discharge plan that addresses risk factors. Thorough documentation enables all parties to focus on the main goal and objective, "The Safety of the Patient and the Safety of the Community."
>
> Don't invest all of your time doing a top-notch clinical risk assessment and then drop the ball on disposition. Communicate with all parties and stay vigilant.

Part Three: Disposition

APPENDIX:

PART ONE

The Clinical Interview

You are not expected to perform the interview in this same sequence. Ultimately, you must explore each domain, but not necessarily in any particular order.

Clinical Disorders

I. Substance Abuse

As with many factors related to suicide, substance abuse troubles us both from a legal standpoint and a clinical standpoint. It is our job to ask the patient if they have been using substances. I always ask this politely, never presumptively - knowing that they are not always likely to tell us the truth. From a legal standpoint, a failure to ask the question could represent malpractice as we fail to consider relevant and available information.

The key to this section of the interview is to demonstrate that you asked the patient about substance abuse. You are not expected to determine if they are telling you the truth, many will not. It is important that you ask about use and document their answers. If you are working in a hospital setting you may have access to drugs of abuse screening. Be sure to ask the patient about any substance that appears in their blood or urine. They may still lie but it is important that you address the result of the screening.

A. Alcohol (ETOH)

I start with alcohol, primarily because alcohol plays a role in so many suicides. Some studies suggest alcohol is on board in 51% of suicides. From my clinical experience, it seems that alcohol is involved in nearly 75% of suicide attempts or people who are threatening suicide. When we look at alcohol, we are first and most primarily concerned about its direct effect on the central nervous system. Alcohol impairs judgment and reduces inhibition. This, clearly, is not helpful in relation to suicide.

If the patient endorses alcohol use, our next step is to warn and advise them. Warn and advise is an important legal position we want to establish. We need to show that we warned the patient about the serious potential side effects or the serious potential effects of substance abuse and we have advised them to seek a chemical dependency evaluation and appropriate chemical dependency treatment. If we fail to do this and the patient takes their life while under the influence of alcohol, you could imagine a scenario in court that would go something like this:

Plaintiff's Attorney says: "Mr. Baer, were you aware that Mr. Smith had a serious alcohol drinking problem?"

I might say, *"No, I wasn't aware."*

Plaintiff's Attorney: "Were you aware that he had alcohol in his system on the day of his suicide?"

"Yes, I was aware of that."

Plaintiff's Attorney: "But you were unaware of his serious drinking problem?"

"That is correct. I was unaware."

Plaintiff's Attorney: "Had you been aware, do you think you would have managed this case differently?"

No matter how you answer this question, you're in trouble. The attorney is leading you down a path that initially seems somewhat benign. Let's imagine that you say, *"No, had I been aware, I would not have managed this case differently."*

Now the attorney can feign shock and say:

Plaintiff's Attorney: "I'm surprised to hear you say that. Your previous testimony established that alcohol plays a role in suicide, numerous research projects establish alcohol plays a role in suicide. It is now your sworn testimony that had you known that this patient had an alcohol abuse problem, you would not have managed this case any differently. Can you tell this Court what other known risk factors did you choose to ignore?"

Clearly, you see by saying "no", you're implying that you don't care about risk factors. Imagine answering it the other way: *"Yes - had I known, I would have managed this case differently."* Plaintiff's attorney now has a clear avenue again.

Plaintiff's Attorney: "I appreciate your honesty in admitting that you should have managed this case differently - because if, in fact, you had known about the alcohol abuse, then the case would have been managed correctly and we would not be in this courtroom today."

No matter how you answer this question you have incriminated yourself. The key to this is the question before: "Were you aware that Mr. Smith had a serious drinking problem?" Your answer there needs to be: *"Yes, I was aware. I warned him and advised him to seek chemical dependency treatment."*

The issue here is one of making an informed decision. The issue is not so much that the patient would have actually taken our advice or the outcome would have actually been any different, but it introduces a question in the jury's mind that had you done your job correctly, had you followed the letter of the law, this patient may, in fact, have taken your advice and sought treatment and wouldn't be dead at this time.

B. Stimulants / Methamphetamine / Amphetamine(s)

Stimulants do not cause as much concern regarding suicide as some other substances but this form of drug abuse is a serious issue that can increase an individual's risk of suicide. Of note is the fact that stimulants can bring about psychosis in prolonged use and psychosis is believed to be the cause of 15% of suicides. However, our main concern related to stimulants is rebound depression. It is not possible to abuse a stimulant without experiencing rebound depression and there is a clear link between depression and suicide. Again, the issue here is warning and advising the patient.

C. Cannabis

Cannabis use is also not closely linked to suicide and the direct effect on the central nervous system does not necessarily increase the patient's odds of taking their life but the detrimental effect of cannabis use should not be minimized.

Some point out that cannabis tends to bring about a lack of motivation and this may be actually protective -it is difficult for me to agree with the protective nature of cannabis but most will agree that cannabis use rarely increases aggressive acts toward self or others. One of my greatest concerns about cannabis is the psychosocial stressors that it introduces into the patient's life. As with any addictive substance or any addictive behavior, the issue of isolation - interpersonal isolation - becomes a concern to us and that is also the concern with prescription abuse.

D. Prescription Abuse

Prescription abuse potentially brings about greater possibilities for psychosocial stressors than even cannabis. The patient who is abusing prescriptions may simply be buying them on the street, but they also may be doctor shopping or altering prescriptions. Also, those who tend to abuse prescription substances, in many cases, have more to lose. They often have more established jobs, more established family relationships and their, "fall from grace" can be considerably greater. This can be referred to as morality shock - a condition that may cause some to be overcome with a sense of shame that they feel they cannot recover from.

E. Substance Abuse Elevating Factors

1. Depression

Potentiating factors related to substance abuse primarily would be depression and interpersonal loss. Many people self medicate their depression by using substances including alcohol. While the patient feels it helps them, in reality they are worsening their depression.

2. Interpersonal Loss

In essence, the whole point of being addicted to a substance is to avoid people. People are not always trustworthy and you cannot always count on them to meet your needs, but substance abusers do count on their substance to meet their needs. Albeit, those needs are not interpersonal, but it's a close approximation that it allows them to withdraw further and further from people and fall deeper and deeper into their substance use. As we know, interpersonal connection - primarily familial connection is our number one protective factor against suicide.

II. Mood Disorders

Mood disorders represent the largest "at risk" patient population. The most common risk factor is depression. In most cases depression is viewed as pathology in and of itself. Depression may merely be an indication that the patient needs to take corrective or protective action in their life.

Imagine a patient walking into a physician's office with acute abdominal pain in the right lower quadrant. A doctor could say: "That could be a lot of things and may be hard to figure it out. Just take these pain pills and check back with me in a month. If it is still hurting we will try a different pill." No physician would treat physical pain in this fashion. Pain is viewed as an indication that something is damaging or out of balance in the patient's life. Pain is an ally as it draws us to the true pathology.

Depression - like pain - is often the patient's ally. This is referred to as state depression as opposed to trait depression which is primarily related to biochemistry rather than events in the patient's life. In the case of state depression it is important to identify the underlying situation that has caused the depression. Until this is discovered and treated the patient will remain at risk for suicide.

It is very important to understand that the brain processes physical pain and emotional pain similarly. In some patients they may experience emotional pain as acutely as others feel physical pain. These patients are clearly at significant risk for suicide.

A. Major Depressive Disorder

Major depression is the number one cause of suicide. 50% - 70% of suicides are thought to be related to major depression. Perhaps if we would all learn to reframe depression and look at it a bit differently, a major depressive episode could actually do more good than harm as we allow it to direct our attention to things that need to be addressed and potentially changed.

Referring back to our "doctor/pain medicine" analogy - we cannot rule out emotional pain because we think it is not an indicator of something bigger. Depression is often a symptom of a larger problem, just like physical pain is a signal pointing to something wrong in the body. Some depression, however appears to simply be the result of an individuals composition rather than an indication of a psych-social stressor.

B. Postpartum Onset

As we're considering depression, we always want to consider postpartum depression. Postpartum depression can lead to suicide though we don't often expect a mother of a newborn to take her life. It is unfortunate but it occasionally happens. In addition to the postpartum depression, we should be concerned about postpartum psychosis. A simple question that can get us into the patient's frame of reference related to postpartum psychosis is: "What do you see in your baby's eyes?" Most moms are going to smile. They're going to say that their baby's eyes are bright, they're intelligent, they have their father's eyes. A mom who is suffering from postpartum depression will often have a flat response. Her eyes don't light up, her affect doesn't change. She simply makes some cursory comment about her baby's eyes being - perhaps - good.

Postpartum psychotic mom, on the other hand, may get nervous. What she often sees in her baby's eyes is malevolence. She thinks that her baby wants to do harm. If you get a nervous response from mom when asked: "What do you see in your baby's eyes?" Follow it up with this next question: "What do you think your baby is thinking?" Most moms would not think their baby was thinking anything. They will look a little bit puzzled. Postpartum psychotic mom may become even more nervous and may, in fact, say, "I really don't want to talk to you. You need to leave. I'm tired now," - because postpartum psychotic mom will often think that her baby is thinking and planning malevolent things; going to kill me, going to kill the children, going to kill my husband. . . . If you get a nervous response from mom on: "What do you see in your baby's eyes?" and "What do you think your baby is thinking?" - dig in for a longer interview and look for postpartum psychosis.

C. Dysthymic Disorder

The issue of dysthymic disorder is not as strongly correlated with suicide as depressive disorder is. Many, many research projects have revealed that depression puts a patients risk at suicide at 10%. Dysthymia is thought to be considerably less. Dysthymia, however, is often related to poor health. So when we think we have discovered dysthymia in a patient, we want to work a little bit harder on getting their physical history.

D. Bipolar Disorder

The issue of bipolar illness is a considerably more important issue. Bipolar patients are thought to take their life at a rate of one in eight. Most of these suicides will occur in the midst of depressive episodes but approximately 15% of bipolar suicides occur in the manic phase. In the case of the manic suicide, it would seem clear that the patient isn't really intending to take their life and we may choose to call that self-inflicted unintentional death; as the patient takes their life in the midst of some grandiose delusion. In some cases, they do intend to end their life, but they believe that they are moving on to a higher or different plane of existence.

A particularly dangerous time for a depressed patient, (either bipolar or uni-polar) is the point at which the depression appears to be resolving and the patients finds the energy and motivation to take their life. It is thought that an antidepressant may improve the patient's motivation, and may increase their energy level before it improves their mood. So while their depression remains the same, they now have energy and motivation to commit suicide. We want to be particularly careful with depressed patients who seem to be rebounding out of a deep trough and especially, our bipolar patients who seem to be rebounding from a serious bout of depression, or recovering from mania and having consequences for their manic behavior.

1. Manic Episode

While most suicides will occur in the depressive phase in the bipolar patient, there are some who will take their life in the manic phase. This is most often in the midst of a grandiose delusion in which they feel invincible or see death as a "transcendence" to another state.

2. Mixed Episode

A mixed patient has mania and depression every day for most of a week. These patients are perhaps some of the most distressed patients we will ever meet; in some cases, even more than your schizophrenia patient - because the bipolar patient often has insight into their illness. They are aware of the nature of their disorder and the mixed nature insures that they are up-and-down on a very frequent basis. They find this incredibly hard to cope with. Many clinicians will mistakenly refer to a mixed episode as a rapid cycler. Rapid cycling is not mixed.

3. Rapid Cycling

A rapid cycling bipolar patient is a patient who has four or more mood episodes in a year. Again, these are very distressed patients. Your average bipolar patient has a mood episode every three years. So four in a year is considerably faster than an average bipolar patient. I consider these patients, the mixed patient and the rapid cycler, to be at highest risk for suicide.

III. Anxiety Disorders

The key to appraising risk in panic disordered patients is to allow them to define severity and their ability to tolerate their symptoms. We cannot objectively define their level of discomfort, this is a subjective feeling that only they can quantify. When they tell us that they can no longer cope with their symptoms we need to provide them with new resources. Always ask the patient if they feel that they need inpatient treatment. Their answer provides the starting point for the disposition of these cases. You are either building an effective outpatient plan that provides both therapy and safety; or you are building a case for admission substantiating imminent risk factors.

A. Panic Attacks

Panic attacks can be one of those "kindling factors" that eventually wear the patient down. In addition, the panic attack may reflect a deeper issue related to trauma/abuse in the patient's life. You need to be very specific with the panic-disordered patient when asking them about their ability to cope. Also be specific regarding their potential abuse of substances, such as prescription benzodiazapines.

Benzodiazapines are tolerance building and habit forming medications, addiction to these medications can occur in the midst of the pre-existing stressors that created the need for the medication prior to the addiction.

B. Agoraphobia

This disorder can often leave a patient feeling ashamed and weak. As with all anxiety disorders, the patient often has insight into their condition; insight can increase the patient distress in some disorders as they feel powerless to overcome behavior that they know to be excessive and unreasonable. If these patients have not engaged in therapy it is important to stress that this condition can be overcome. For those who have been in therapy but state that it does not help you need to consider the possibility that their condition may be related to personality disorders and less related to a clinical condition. It is important to note that a patient who has earnestly engaged in unsuccessful therapy may conclude that their situation is truly hopeless. You will need to consider an inpatient stay so this patient can develop a therapy plan they have confidence in.

C. Obsessive-Compulsive Disorder

This is a very challenging disorder that has many facets of risk to consider. We first address the most obvious stressor, the patient's level of distress. Then we want to consider the particular theme that their obsessions take as well as the nature of the compulsions. Some themes such as the fear that you may assault someone or commit a sexual crime can be very distressing and the patient may take their life to prevent this from happening. Some compulsions are so disruptive that the patient feels that a "normal" life is impossible and they elect to end their life rather than suffer the frustration and possible feelings of shame they may be experiencing.

D. Post-Traumatic Stress Disorder

The base rate for civilian PTSD is reported to be 3%. It is likely that this estimate is too low. Many people suffer from PTSD. The most common cause is interpersonal violence ranging from domestic violence to a random sexual assault.

It is helpful to view this disorder in a slightly different view. It appears that these patients suffer from continued "rehearsal" as their mid brain causes them to re-experience the traumatic event again and again. The purpose of this rehearsal is to prepare them for the next time they encounter a similar situation. This becomes exhausting and overwhelming. In some cases therapy makes this worse because the therapist over activates the patients emotional centers during a session. While all PTSD patients are at risk for suicide, those who enter into therapy may be at higher risk if the therapy is not going well.

IV. Schizophrenia And Other Psychotic Disorders

A. Life-Time Risk For Suicide

Schizophrenia patients have a 10% lifetime risk of suicide. Psychosis accounts for 10 - 15% of all suicides.

Suicide is the number one cause of premature death in psychotic patients. In the case of schizophrenia, positive symptoms such as paranoid delusions represent the higher risk patients while negative symptoms such as blunted affect and lack of motivation may actually reduce risk as they lack the motivation to take their life. It would never be advisable however to dismiss the risk of suicide in a patient who primarily displayed the negative symptoms of schizophrenia.

B. Positive Symptoms

All schizophrenia patients have significant suicide risk; patients who predominantly have positive symptoms have the highest risk. Consider a patient who suffers from "ideas of reference." They feel that everyone is talking about them or looking at them. It is as if they are the only naked person in every room and they are forced every day to face that degree of discomfort. Eventually they lose resilience and their will to live. Other patients believe that they may be kidnapped and tortured or that they possess knowledge that will end the world. The variations on delusions cannot be predicted but we can recognize the significant role these delusions play in suicide.

C. Negative Symptoms

It is never wise to assume that a particular patient group is safe but it is accurate to conclude that negative symptoms may make a schizophrenia patient safer because they lack the energy and in some cases the ability to take their life.

D. Elevating Factors Of The Paranoid Patient

It is important to ask the patient with paranoid delusions: "What might you have to do to protect yourself?" Some patients with more passive traits may say, "Nothing." or "I might have to kill myself." Other patients with more aggressive traits may indicate that they may harm others in self-defense. I generally always ask: *Could you ever hurt another person to protect yourself or others?*"

While the concept of self-defense seems reasonable to most people the true issue here is the perception of a threat when there is no true threat. You should also ask; *"Would you ever take your life to escape those who you feel are after you?"* Some paranoid individuals fear the potential method of death more than actual death and they would rather die in a manner of their choosing rather than wait in fear.

E. Elevating Factors For Schizophrenia And Psychotic Disorders

1. Depressive Symptoms

The schizoaffective patient may represent some of the highest risk patients we will ever see. This combination of schizophrenia and affective disorder can be very complicated to treat. This is especially true in the case of the bipolar type-schizoaffective patient.

2. Formerly High-Functioning

These patients may retain enough insight to recognize the severity of their loss.

3. Young Age

In general this risk factor applies to males as men develop schizophrenia approximately 10 younger than women. Schizophrenia tends to emerge in the early 20s for men and 30s for women.

4. Early Stage Of Illness

Like the formerly high functioning patient, this patient may retain enough insight to recognize the severity of their loss.

5. Improvement / Relapse Cycle

Again, the issue here is recognizing the severity of loss.

V. Schizoaffective Disorder

This patient is extremely challenging to manage. Their combination of affective symptoms combined with either positive or negative aspects of schizophrenia puts them at unique risk.

A. Bipolar Type

Mania combined with psychosis typically presenting in the form of a grandiose delusion can cause the patient to take their life unintentionally as they may believe that they cannot actually die or that their death may be temporary. In addition, mania combined with paranoia may cause them to take their life in a defensive effort; in some cases they do not view death as final. This may be because they believe they can "get a new body" or they may see themselves as invincible.

B. Depressive Type

Again, we never assume any patient is safe but this patient is generally considered safer than the bipolar type-schizoaffective patient. Loss of motivation and psycho-motor retardation seem to be protective. However, never assume that any particular symptom indicates safety merely by its presence.

VI. Delusional Disorders

I believe that delusions are elaborate ego defense mechanisms. Ego defense mechanisms distort reality. We all need to distort reality occasionally but the delusional patient incorporates their ego defense mechanism into the foundation of their life. These delusions can be very resilient and therefore difficult to modify or treat. We need to evaluate their potential behavior within the context of their delusion.

A. Erotomanic type

The erotomanic patient believes that someone is in love with them. This patient is more likely to engage in stalking rather than homicide or suicide. We simply ask this patient about their thoughts regarding violence. Male erotomanic patients are more likely to be violent but females are more likely to suffer from this delusion.

Of particular note is triangulation. In triangulation the delusional patient sees someone standing between them and the object of their delusion such as a spouse or significant other. They may believe that if this person was removed the object of their delusion would be free to profess their love.

B. The Grandiose Type

The grandiose patient believes they have a special power, ability or perhaps a special relationship with deity. They may take their life in the belief that they have been called to sacrifice themselves, or they are being called to a higher "plane or purpose".

C. The Jealous Type

Keeping within the context of ego defense mechanism, I first consider if this patient is using the delusional system as a deflection from their own feelings or fears of sexual inadequacy. Claiming that your partner is sexually unfaithful is the perfect smoke screen to hide behind if you do not want to be sexually intimate for any number of reasons. If you suspect this is the reason for the delusional system you should not confront this as you may increase the risk of suicide in the event this ego defense collapses. This particular defense should only be confronted within a well establish therapeutic alliance. If the delusion appears to be genuine there is a risk of homicide if the patient feels they know who their partner is being unfaithful with. We must always specifically ask if the patient is thinking of harming himself or herself, their partner, or the individual they feel their partner is involved with.

D. Persecutory Type

The persecutory patient clearly has a touch of paranoia. Perhaps they don't perform threat appraisal well and therefore cannot adequately find a sense of peace in social settings, perhaps they have attracted the attention of someone who actually does want to harm them.

These patients will often choose someone who is fairly innocuous to focus their anxiety on. They may also choose a nebulous "class" of people such as "Satan worshipers". This gives them an "anxiety sink" of sorts - a place to focus their otherwise free floating and overwhelming fear. It is important to ask these patients: "What might you have to do to protect yourself?" If their temperament is somewhat aggressive they may be at risk for violence. If they are fearful enough they may be at risk for suicide.

E. Somatic Type

This patient is concerned that there is something wrong with their body. In some cases they may take lethal action, as they fear the delusion more than death. This may be due to the belief that they will experience a particularly painful death or perhaps they fear that they carry some disease that puts others or perhaps the entire world at risk.

VII. Eating Disorders

These patients face the dual risk of the devastating physical effects of their disorder as well as the emotional burdens that may have caused their disorder. Attempting to address this disorder in the midst of a crisis is not likely to lead to a good outcome and can intensify the crisis. It is generally best to work from the research driven hypotheses that these disorders arise out of a need for a sense of control in the anorexic patient, and perhaps both control and a need to punish ones self in bulimia.

This need for both control and self-punishment is often rooted in a history of sexual abuse. Suicide risk can persist for decades following sexual abuse as the lingering victim effects cause more and more relationship damage. Eventually a sense of hopelessness and a need to escape may overwhelm them.

I never pursue the issue of sexual abuse in the midst of a crisis. I identify it and communicate a sense of hope regarding resolution of the issues but I do not want to discuss the trauma as that will almost certainly add energy to the current crisis.

Keep in mind that many of these patients have attempted therapy several times with limited or no success. Because of this I never give trivial advice, nor do I act as if this can be quickly fixed. I generally tell them that I am aware of the complexity of the issues and I assure them that current research indicates that recovery is possible with a skilled therapist who proves to be a good match for them.

VIII. Insomnia

Primary insomnia, or insomnia that is not related to another disorder, can be extremely frustrating at the least and may cause extreme distress. It is important to note that insomnia can be an independent predictor of increased suicide risk. This means that even when there is no other mental illness present patients with insomnia have an increased risk of suicide attempts.

IX. Personality Disorders

Personality disordered patients can be the most challenging patients you will evaluate. By definition, personality disorders consist of an enduring set of maladaptive characteristics that guide the patient in nearly every interaction in life. The challenge for you is to determine what elements of risk are chronic and what elements may be acute.

Simply asking the patient what has recently changed in their life is generally the best way to identify current, acute stressors. You may also ask: "What have you done to manage situations like this in the past?" If they have never encountered, or successfully managed their current situation you will need to be especially careful. Personality disordered patients do take their life in spite of the common belief that they just make threats.

A. Borderline Personality Disorder / Features

Clearly, the borderline patient is the most frequently evaluated personality disordered patient. These patients have chronic suicide risk. For some, this is their primarily "engagement style". It is how they insure that others give them attention and energy. For others, they genuinely struggle with thoughts of suicide.

The patient who uses suicide as a means to engage with others will frequently report multiple attempts, sometimes over 20. The actual risk with these patients will be small but they must be treated as if they are genuinely at risk or they may attempt to "validate" their risk with an attempt. I generally act as if I am going to quickly hospitalize these patients. In many cases this is more than they wanted and they will begin to withdraw the threat. As a rule, I keep the pressure on long enough to cause a bit of discomfort in order to deter them from using this as a manipulative strategy in the future. This may prevent repeat visits by reinforcing a consequence for their words and actions.

I tell these patients that it is my job to insure their safety and if they cannot assure me that they are safe I have to take responsibility for keeping them safe. In reality, it is rarely advisable, nor therapeutic to hospitalize these patients, many psychiatrists will refuse to admit these patients. My goal here is to reduce the secondary gain they receive from making threats. They are looking for "energy" from me and I give them consequence instead.

All this has to be done without giving them any emotional energy at all. If they sense that you are extremely concerned for them, angered or annoyed, they have achieved their goal. They simply want energy. I want them to feel appropriate professional detachment with a simple and single goal; their current safety.

1. Elevated Risk Factors For The Borderline Patient

a. Mental Disorder

Nearly every borderline patient has a concurrent psychological disorder such as Posttraumatic Stress Disorder or Depression. When the symptoms seem to be at the forefront of the current crisis I generally act as if they do not have a personality disorder and I focus on the mental health condition.

An example of this may be the patient with PTSD who is experiencing more flashbacks or other re-experiencing symptoms then usual. This takes us back to the question: "What has recently changed, or what is new?"

b. Substance Abuse

Many borderline patients have substance abuse problems. We need to be particularly alert for recent and significant psycho/social changes as a result of the abuse, such as a patient who may be loosing custody of their children due to their substance use. In addition, the added impulsivity of alcohol abuse must be considered though this impulsivity is especially hard to manage or treat.

c. Previous Attempts

Nearly all borderline patients have previous attempts. Pay particular attention to determining the severity of the attempt and their need for medical attention. Also determine if the attempts are generally impulsive or planned. While it is nearly impossible to mitigate the risk represented by impulsivity, you can intervene more effectively with the patients who plan their attempts.

Also be aware of secondary gain for the borderline who make a serious suicide attempt while on an inpatient unit. Screen for weapons.

B. Antisocial Personality Disorder / Features

Some clinicians feel that Antisocial personalities are too self consumed to kill themselves. This is not a safe position to take. Antisocial personality disordered patients do take their lives, especially as they approach middle age.

Stanton Samenow, perhaps the best researcher and author on this personality disorder suggests that as this patient's anger and frustration with the world grows, so does their suicide risk.

1. Elevated Risk Factors For Antisocial Personality Disorder

Concurrent Mental Health Disorder:
Like the borderline patient, many of these patients have other underlying mental health conditions. I always assign risk to the mental health conditions issues first. This means that I treat the risk as acute rather than chronic.

C. Narcissistic Personality Disorder/ Features

The Narcissist is often viewed in the same light at the Antisocial, too self absorbed to take their life, again, this is false and a dangerous position to take. In particular, these patients are at risk in the midst of the "narcissistic wound syndrome." This wound occurs when they have suffered public failure, humiliation or criticism. These patients are also at higher risk as they age.

Medical Problems

There is little research to indicate that any particular medical problem uniquely contributes to suicide. Many illnesses cause sufficient distress to motivate thoughts of suicide. Some illnesses such as Multiple Sclerosis and Alzheimer's disease directly affect the brain in ways that may contribute to suicide risk.

In general we are concerned about the patient's opinion of their physical health and their thoughts regarding a course of action. Some patients have very low pain tolerance and find the prospect of a painful illness far more than they can cope with. In other cases the idea of being dependent on others for such basic tasks as bathing or dressing is overwhelming from either a human dignity standpoint or a fear of becoming a burden. In addition, some are concerned about the cost of protracted health care and an unwillingness to leave loved ones with little or no money after the patient has passed away.

Psychosocial Stressors

It is not possible to rate psychosocial risk factors. The best we can do is to inquire about these risk factors and assess the impact the stressor has on the patient. Only the patient can assign "value" to a risk factor. It should be noted that it is these current stressors that generally serve as the catalyst for the act of suicide. If we were using fire triangle (ignition, fuel, oxygen) as an analogy we would consider the psycho/social stressor to be the match that ignites the fuel.

The most common stressor is the loss of a relationship. Keep in mind that some people experience the emotional pain of loss as acutely as others feel physical pain. These patients may find the "pain of loneliness" as Jonathan Cacioppo calls it, unbearable. Others are overwhelmed by financial stressors to include the loss of a job and perhaps everything they own. It is our job to determine if any of these losses have completely overwhelmed their coping mechanisms.

Psychotic Violence Inquiry

It is important to note that most people who are mentally ill are not violent. They are in fact more likely to be victims of violence rather than perpetrators of violence.

To get a sense of perspective lets look at some statistics from the National Institute of Mental Health. The lifetime prevalence for committing an act of violence against someone is 7% for the general population. For those who abuse substances it is 35%. For those who have a mental illness it is 16%. For those who abuse substances and have a mental illness is it 44%. Clearly the most predictive factor is the use of drugs and alcohol.

There are however several factors that have been identified as indicators of impending violence when assessing individuals with mental illnesses. As always, it is important to state that it is **never** possible to determine what a person will **not** do. It is possible to recognize known factors associated with violent acts. We should first determine if the patient is currently being treated and if they are treatment compliance. A lack of compliance alone may be reason enough to detain a patient especially if they have a history of violence.

I. History

History, as always, is our starting point when assessing possible violent behavior. Have they committed a violent act in the past? What were the circumstances of that violent act? Was there provocation involved or perceived provocation? Does this current situation mirror the prior violent acts in any way? When we are aware of violence in the past we need to ask the patient about the incident or incidents and allow them to give us a sense of their perspective. This helps us determine the likelihood that they will react with violence again.

II. Stated Intent

In many cases a psychotic patient will make no attempt to hide their violent intentions or actions. This lack of insight is one of the factors forensic psychologists use to determine if someone is fit to stand trial. As a rule, any attempt to hide ones actions indicates a lack of mental illness. When you do not have the insight to hide your violent intention or action it is a strong indicator of mental illness. Simply asking a psychotic patient if they intend to commit a violent act will often yield very useful information. Sometimes they will make generic threats such as "I am going to kill the next person who tries to read my mind." Other times there is "attribution". They "attribute" evil intent to someone and then announce their intention to harm that person. We will almost always have to act in the case of attribution.

III. Delusions

Fixed false beliefs often become the foundation for violent behavior. Violence follows two broad paths in these cases. The first path is where the patient feels someone or something is going to harm them. They may take defensive action that leads to violence or in some cases they may take their own life rather be than subjected to what they believe will be torture.

The other path involves the belief that they need to protect the world or someone else from evil. This may require them to kill a potential perpetrator or it may involve them killing someone they believe will be a victim of something worse than death. In either case the patient will often reveal their intention if we ask in a non-threatening manner.

IV. Personality Disorders

The Cluster B personality disorders (borderline, narcissistic, histrionic, and antisocial) all have elevated risk for violence. This is especially true in the case of the antisocial who is most likely to commit a violent act for personal gain. The borderline and the narcissist are more likely to commit acts of violence impulsively or for retribution.

PART TWO

Specific Risk Inquiry: Suicide

Much of the information you gain here is simply an act of "due diligence". You are demonstrating that you have sought out relevant and available information so that you can make an informed decision. Some of the information will not be of tremendous clinical value; it may simply have legal value in the event you have to defend your disposition in the event of a bad outcome.

I. Recent History of Suicide Attempts:

A. Suicide Attempts

A previous history of suicide attempts is a significant predictor of future attempts but is also an overvalued predictor. Half of all completed suicides occur on the first attempt. 55% of males who kill themselves do so on their first attempt. 45% of female suicides occur on their first attempt. Clearly this means that in half of all suicides there was no previous suicide attempt to alert the clinician to the seriousness of the patients' suicidal intent.

Suicide attempts fall into two broad categories - painful ways to die and painless ways to die. I believe that the nature of the suicide attempt has some predictive value regarding likelihood of future attempts. Patients who attempt suicide in what is perceived as a painless way such as an overdose are often suffering from what Edwin Schniedman refers to as psychache. This is a condition in which an individual suffers intolerable pain experienced at the very core of their sense of self. I believe these patients are trying to end their suffering in as painless of a way as possible. They do not want to add to their suffering, but end it.

Patients who attempt suicide in more painful ways such as cutting, hanging, drowning, hypothermia or any number of other methods will often report that they were attempting to punish themselves in death with the hope that God would allow them into heaven. They often view their suicide as a sort of self-imposed purgatory. These patients often have some hidden "sin" that they feel they must atone for. I believe that these patients represent higher risk for future attempts. Their need to punish themselves is not likely to go away as this need tends to have fairly deep roots often involving abuses perpetrated against them or abuses they have perpetrated against others.

I will offer suggestions regarding possible motivation for each type of suicide but it is a mistake to interpret a person's behavior without allowing them to explain their motivation. I always ask the following question. "What were your thoughts regarding the method you chose?" This is not a leading question nor does it attempt to explain their possible motivation. In some cases, the patient has not given thought to why they chose a particular method. This question will give them an opportunity to consider their own actions. Make no effort to rush this answer nor should you give them suggestions if they appear unable to answer.

B. Methods

1. Overdose

I believe that the overdose most often represents the patient who is looking for a painless way to end their suffering. While these patients can certainly be at risk for repeat attempts we can infer that if their emotional pain is addressed their need to die will be diminished.

2. Cutting

Death via exsanguination is rare - accounting for only 2% of suicides. Though it is certainly possible to die in this manner, our bodies like to hold on to our blood and nature has many tricks to prevent death due to blood loss.

Clearly this manner of suicide is more violent and painful than an overdose. It often carries with it a significant degree of self-hatred and/or a need to punish oneself for perceived sins or faults. If I were conducting long-term therapy I would attempt to get at the root of what drives this violent type of attempt. I feel that the patient's risk of future attempts is high until they have an opportunity to resolve these underlying issues.

Parasuicide:

An act where intended outcome is not death.

Parasuicide is the strongest indicator for a future suicide attempt. Half of those who commit suicide have a history of parasuicide.

49

3. Hanging

Hanging appears to be significantly motivated by self hatred - even more so than the cutting patient. Again, I am concerned about the underlying motivation. I want to understand what drives this need for punishment and "atonement" within the act of suicide. I feel this is crucial if we are to prevent future suicide attempts.

4. Shooting

While a gun is a violent means of death it can also be a painless one. Only the patient can reveal their motivation regarding this method of death. Clearly, you will interview very few patients who have attempted suicide via gunshot as this method rarely fails. I have conducted a number of interviews with individuals who claim that the gun misfired, I am very skeptical of misfires. I consider most of these patients to be attention seeking though I never confront them on this issue. Guns rarely misfire, either the entire story is a fabrication or they didn't load the gun. In cases where they failed to load the gun it may be that they were "rehearsing" their suicide. As a rule, I hospitalize anyone who reports a suicide attempt with a gun even if I feel it was an attention seeking strategy.

5. Automobile Accident

Auto accident suicide attempts are often associated with people who wanted their suicide to look like an accident. This may be for insurance purposes or to avoid causing guilt in family members or an attempt to protect their "legacy" within the family. In other cases the auto accident suicide was an impulsive act.

6. Carbon Monoxide Poisoning / Car Gassing

This method is often viewed as a quiet, painless option. It is not nearly as successful as it used to be due to catalytic converters on cars, in some cases it takes 10 times longer to reach a lethal carbon monoxide level in newer vehicles.

C. Is Medical Care Needed?

This question is intended to give you a sense of lethality of both the patient's intent and method. Suicide attempts that would have been lethal without medical intervention are viewed as the most serious but in an assessment sense they are no more serious than the attempt that was believed to be lethal but was not. Both patient groups are in need of significant intervention.

D. Discovered By:

One of the most important elements to consider regarding attempts is who found the patient. I believe the most predictive data is revealed in how the patient's attempt was discovered. Was there a "staged rescue" in which the patient clearly intended for their attempt to be discovered or was it truly a "random find" in which someone happens to come upon the patient in the midst of their suicide attempt. The apparent "random find" intervention probably represents our highest risk patient. We need to ask them how they feel about being alive. Are they upset with whoever found them? Do they believe that the intervention means they "have a purpose to go on living?" Do they still want to die?

Some patients actually seem to benefit from the suicide attempt; it forces them to reappraise their life as they discover meaning and value in previously unappreciated areas. They will insist that they would never attempt suicide again. Occasionally you may be tempted to discharge these patients from the medical floor, I think this is a mistake. They have not received a full psychiatric evaluation nor has an appropriate treatment plan been put in place. The argument that they "learned their lesson" will appear extremely weak in the spotlight of litigation.

The staged rescue patient is clearly intending to manipulate others. If they have been successful with this in the past this will likely become a "learned behavior" they incorporate into their life. If the manipulative attempt does not control others they may reject this as a strategy, or they may increase the perceived lethality of the attempt in an attempt to force others to "take them seriously". You will need to invest the time and energy needed to determine what path they are most likely to pursue.

Your response to the patient who appears to be manipulative needs to be strong and consistent. You will always treat this patient as if they truly intended to take their life. Discuss with them the full range of interventions available including inpatient and outpatient options. Let them know the possibility of involuntary hospitalization exists. You don't want this to seem like a threat, you simply want them to know where this behavior is heading if it persists. If they did truly intend to take their life you want them to be aware of all treatment possibilities, if they didn't really intend to take their life they will perhaps develop other affiliation strategies if the potential of involuntary hospitalization does not appeal to them. **See Disposition section for further discussion.**

II. Remote History of Suicide Attempts:

Suicide attempts that took place a number of years ago may or may not have clinical significance but they always have legal significance. Your primary task regarding remote history of suicide attempts is to demonstrate that you were aware of that history and the patient's reaction to their previous attempt. Your failure to document previous attempts will be catastrophic in the event of a lawsuit.

Plaintiff's attorney will first ask you if you were aware of any previous attempts, when you say that you were not, the attorney will then ask if you are aware that a previous history of suicide is a significant predictor of future attempts. You have to indicate that you were aware of this or the attorney has already demonstrated that you are not competent to perform a suicide risk assessment. After the attorney has established that previous attempts indicate increased risk, and after the attorney has established that you were not aware of this risk you will then be asked if you would have managed the case differently if you had been aware of the patient's previous attempt. You are already in serious trouble for failing to inquire about previous risk and you are now about to slip a noose around your neck no matter how you answer the question. If you say you would not have managed the case differently you will then be asked what other risk factors you choose to ignore. If you say you would have managed the case differently you will be thanked for your honestly as you have just admitted that you mismanaged the case and that mismanagement resulted in a suicide.

The only way out of this trap is be aware of all previous attempts, or more correctly you need to demonstrate that you inquired about recent and remote suicide attempts. If the patient lied to you and failed to tell you about previous attempts, no malpractice occurred. If you failed to inquire, malpractice may have occurred. This is an easy situation to avoid, make sure this question is asked and answered, and of course documented. It is also important to ask any possible collateral sources such as family members if they are aware of any previous attempts with this patient.

A. Multiple Attempts

Multiple attempts generally indicate a borderline personality disorder.

B. Severity Of Attempts

1. Gesture Versus Actual Intent

Some suicide attempts clearly appear to be a gesture rather than a genuine attempt at suicide. It is important to document the gesture in a way that supports a possible outpatient treatment plan rather than hospitalization.

An example of a gesture may be someone who takes 5 Xanax tablets when the bottle contains significantly more. When I ask the patient how many pills they took I always ask if there were more pills in the bottle. If they say there were more pills I never ask "why didn't you take them all?" Asking "why" often puts people on the defensive. I ask, *"What were your thoughts regarding the quantity of pills you took?"* This is neither leading nor perceived as a challenge. It is a simple inquiry into their state of mind. If they give me an answer that leads me to believe the attempt was genuine I move on to other questions. If they give me an answer that is not convincing I then follow up with "Do you think you intended to die or do you just need people to know how much pain you are in?"

When documenting the gesture I generally write; *This patient's action implied gesture rather than true intent, when asked 'Did you really want to die or do you just need people to know how much you hurt', the patient replied, 'No one takes me seriously, I had to do something to get their attention.'*

In the borderline patient any suggestion that we do not take their gesture seriously is likely to cause them to "up the ante". It is my belief that many borderline patients kill themselves accidentally as they attempt to prove how suicidal they are.

We are all born with the innate ability to manipulate others. Manipulation, or indirect communication is our native tongue. As infants our survival depended on our ability to successfully manipulate our caregivers to meet our every need. Our first manipulative tool is pain. We demonstrate that we are in pain by crying and we inflict pain on our caregivers by crying. Pain becomes common ground upon which the attachment relationship begins. Perhaps this is why people care so much about sharing their pain with others. It provides a foundation upon which a trusting relationship can be built.

Most people never truly outgrow this strategy. They continue to base their relationships with others on pain. Suicide is often seen as the ultimate expression of emotional pain as well as a painful thing you can "inflict" on those who have displeased you. It is within this context that many suicide threats occur.

2. Dangerous / Not Lethal / Believed To Be Lethal

A key question in interviewing patients who have attempted suicide is, "Did you believe your actions would end your life?" This is far more important to you than the actual lethality of their actions. Many patients believe that over the counter (OTC) sleeping medications can kill them. This is not always true. They, however may have had the genuine expectation that death would have been the result.

A common less than lethal overdose is anxiety medication or benzodiazapines. These medications are typically only lethal when taken in combination with other drugs such as opiates, narcotics or barbiturates. Alcohol will also make these anxiety medications lethal. Fortunately, many patients are unaware of the need for a poly-substance overdose.

3. Dangerous / Potentially Lethal Or Lethal Without Intervention

In both cases you clearly act as if the attempt was genuine even in those cases when you suspect the patient "staged a rescue." You have no choice but to act as if the patient fully intended to die, in most cases regarding lethal or nearly lethal means the patient did intend to die or at the least had significant ambivalence regarding death. The highest level of intervention is called for even if the patient now states they want to live.

III. Current Suicidal Ideation:

There is a significant difference between suicidal ideation and suicidal intent. We want to identify both. The patient with suicidal ideation needs intervention specifically targeted at the source of their discomfort. This may require both medication and psychotherapy. The patient who identifies both ideation and intent needs very active intervention. It is likely that an inpatient option may have to be explored.

A. Passive Thoughts

Some clinicians will say that everyone has had thoughts of suicide. If this is true then most people have had passive thoughts of suicide rather than active thoughts. When you ask this patient if they have ever considered suicide they reply "Yeah, I have thought of it but I could never do it." They have no plan nor do they have intent. This is a patient that rarely requires inpatient intervention. It is important to document that they know how to receive help if their passive thoughts become active and they begin to consider a plan.

B. Active Thoughts

This patient is actively considering suicide; they may or may not have a plan but they have clearly moved beyond simply considering suicide. It is important to determine if this patient is conflicted regarding suicide or if they experience a sense of peace regarding death.

This distinction between "egosyntonic" (meaning they find this idea peaceful and it aligns with their personal goals) and "egodystonic" (meaning they are disturbed by this idea) thoughts of suicide is very important when attempting to assign risk to the possibility of suicide. Clearly, the egosyntonic patient carries the higher risk.

C. Are They Able To Control Their Suicidal Thoughts?

Persistent and obsessive suicidal ideation clearly represents significant danger to the patient. Again, attempt to determine if the thoughts are egosyntonic or egodystonic.

D. Have They Made Preparations For Death?

I have seen elaborate preparations for death that were simply histrionic attempts to gain attention and control others. I have also seen subtle preparations for death that only a family member could notice and interpret correctly. It is important to consider collateral sources of information regarding this topic.

E. Are They Experiencing Command Hallucinations?

Command hallucinations can present a difficult legal position for us. Keeping in mind that juries are made up of people off the street, the average person has no idea how common it is for schizophrenia patients to hear voices. In many cases these patients have had voices telling them to kill themselves for years. How then do we know when to intervene? In general I am looking for three things. The first is a change in the voice either in quality of the voice or content of the message. Second, research reveals that a "kind benevolent voice" is more likely to be followed, keep in mind it is quality of the voice at issue here, not the content of the message. Third, I want the patient to appear confident when they tell me that they will not follow the command.

F. Content of suicidal ideation:

1. Ambivalence

Disposition for the ambivalent patient can be challenging. They generally do not qualify for inpatient services as they do not generally have an active and or imminent plan. Our best option with this patient is to establish a full range of necessary intervention services to include treatment for substance use and dependence. We then ask them to commit to utilizing these services. In addition, we insure that they are aware of crisis intervention services and establish that they both know how to access these services and are willing to do so in the event that they are feeling actively suicidal.

In an ideal world the patient will promise to get treatment and they will also promise to seek crisis intervention rather than take their life. In the real world patients often refuse all efforts at intervention and refuse to promise to call crisis services. As a rule, this patient does not qualify for a civil commitment and they clearly do not qualify for a voluntary inpatient stay. What then do we do?

You need to first establish that they are not suffering from a serious and debilitating mental illness. In effect, you are saying they are rational and qualified to make treatment choices, even if they make bad treatment choices. You then establish that the patient is aware of all community resources. You then establish that you have "warned the patient" about the possibility of suicide if they refuse services. I always conclude with the statement that "this patient has been strongly advised to seek services."

2. Psychological Pain

Does time heal all wounds? Clearly it does not. Some emotional pain is so pervasive and or acute that the patient is completely overwhelmed by it. This patient is not as committed to death as they are desperate for relief. If a reasonable plan for resolution of their emotional pain can be presented this patient may be deterred from their suicidal path. If not, admission should be strongly considered.

3. Hopelessness

It is important to ask patients "What have you done to try to resolve this problem?" Patients feel hopeless when they have exhausted all avenues of resolution available to them, or all avenues they have considered. It is our job to broaden their horizon and point out other avenues of resolution. Edwin Shneidman refers to this as addressing the problem of "constriction". Their pain has so constricted their view that they cannot imagine other options.

4. A History Of Sexual Abuse

Individuals who have suffered childhood sexual abuse often suffer from a range of chronic "victim effects." Perhaps the most common is a sense of guilt and shame as children often feel complicit in the sexual activity. This sense of complicity comes from a few sources. First, children are very egocentric; they naturally assume that everything is about them and for them. In addition, perpetrators often tell the child it is their fault. Children nearly always believe "grown ups".

A significant source of guilt and confusion is found in fact that children almost always "freeze" in response to sexual abuse. Freeze is the first "F" in the 3 "F"s of panic. Freeze, fight, flight. Children almost universally freeze when confronted with life threatening trauma, freeze is the most adaptive response for a child. In addition to freeze, they generally go mute, also a protective, adaptive response. This autonomic reaction to sexual abuse causes significant confusion as the child fails to understand that these behaviors are beyond their control. The perpetrator often reinforces the guilt and shame by pointing out to the child that they failed to take protective action and therefore must have enjoyed the contact or at the least were complicit.

This childhood foundation of confusion, guilt and shame is carried into adult life. Nearly every intimate relationship the individual has occurs within the shadow of this abuse. Even consensual sexual intimacy within the context of a loving relationship can have echoes of exploitation and shame. Eventually these victims of childhood abuse lose the will and strength to keep living.

This can especially be true when the perpetrator is someone whom the victim would have reasonably expected to protect and provide for them. Children have the "*a priori*" assumption that caregivers are infallible and omnipotent. It doesn't occur to children that caregivers can be wrong, or do wrong. This makes it very difficult for children to correctly assign blame to caregivers who abuse them. This *a priori* assumption often persists into adult life as we see adult victims of childhood sexual abuse still living with a sense of guilt and shame. It appears that they would rather carry the responsibility for the abuse rather than accept that their caregiver was wrong. Perhaps the idealized view of the infallible and omnipotent caregiver is more comforting than any version of actual truth that shatters this illusion.

Notes:

_____

_____

_____

_____

_____

_____

_____

_____

_____

_____

IV. Evaluating Suicidal Intent:

A. No Intent But Not Able To "Contract" For Safety.

It is important to note that contracts for safety are an old, outdated and useless tool in crisis intervention; this is discussed in another section (p. 88). The patient who cannot or will not insure their safety comes in two varieties, clinical disorders and personality disorders.

The clinical patient is generally making an honest statement about their inability to promise that they will not take their life. Many will state that they hope they don't kill themselves but they can't be sure that they won't. These patients generally should be hospitalized. If not, there needs to be a solid crisis plan in place and a good reason to believe that the patient will utilize that plan in the event of overwhelming suicidal ideation.

The personality disordered patient is generally being manipulative. Your response to this patient will vary according to your familiarity with the patient and your available resources. I generally pursue an inpatient disposition with these patients in spite of the fact that research suggests that inpatient stays are not productive.

This patient generally presents in one of these two following ways. The first patient doesn't want admission but does want people to invest energy in them over the next several days. The second group is seeking admission but it is clearly manipulative. With both patients groups I generally push for admission.

In the case of the patient who simply wants others to be worried about them, I inform them that no one wants to be more worried about their life than they are. If they can't insure their own safety it is unreasonable to ask others to do it for them. I explain that an admission is the only reasonable course of action.

In the case of the patient who seems to simply be manipulating in order to obtain a bed I am trying to avoid the possibility that the patient will escalate their manipulative behavior if I deny them that bed. In this case I always suggest that the treating psychiatrist makes the patient stay as stark and unrewarding as possible.

B. Suicidal Intent Related To:

1. Wish To Die

Most often this patient will feel intense suffering of some sort and they will want to end that suffering in a fairly painless way. Offering them realistic solutions or treatment is your best option.

2. Desire To Hurt Someone Else

This will likely be a revenge suicide that is intended to cause someone else to feel responsible for the death. These suicides tend to be violent and dramatic and most often carried out by teens or adults with personality disorders

3. Need To Escape

Anticipation is a powerful force in our lives and negative anticipation may be more than some people can tolerate. These patients need help coming to terms with actual or possible frightening or painful changes in their life. In some cases they have already suffered significant consequences and do not feel they can bear the long term results.

4. Need To Punish Self

I am always concerned when someone feels they have done such a bad thing that they need to die. I believe that we have to get the patient to "confess" this perceived "capital offense" or they will eventually take their life. Push gently, most of these patients need inpatient care and there is limited value to deep disclosure in an assessment setting.

It is important to remember that psychotic patients will often experience delusional guilt sufficient enough to cause this type of suicide. As with most psychotic suicides, it is likely to be a very violent death.

C. Suicidal Plan:

Inquiring about a suicide plan is primarily a matter of "due diligence". We are gathering information to make an "informed decision" regarding a disposition. Some clinicians use the presence of a plan or the absence of a plan as the defining criteria when attempting to determine risk is present. I weigh this data, but rarely assign significant power to it. Sometimes the plan seems elaborate and even grandiose, in these cases I may feel that genuine risk is not present and the patient is primarily attempting to manipulate others. In other cases I have seen patients who are vague or even deny a suicide plan yet they are in fact suicidal.

D. Impulsivity

Impulsivity is not necessarily a treatable condition; therefore identifying it is of questionable value. This information can however be useful when you are uncertain of a disposition and you need something to push you one way or the other. In cases where you are uncertain, allow the presence of impulsivity to push you towards an inpatient disposition.

A possible strategy with impulsive patients is to ask them to write a series of notes if they do decide to take their life. Try to have at least 3 people on this list. The hope is that in the process of writing the notes they will experience a cathartic release while allowing the impulse to dissipate. Patients are more likely to agree to this rather than agreeing to call us when they plan to take their life. Writing the notes has an egosyntonic feel to it as it is a step towards their goal rather than a step away. In the event they abandon their suicide plan after writing the notes, ask them to give the notes to a therapist. This reveals insight into their state of mind and will also force them to write new notes if they become suicidal in the future.

E. Thoughts Regarding Their Future

The patient's perception of their future can be very useful especially when you are considering an outpatient disposition.

1. Faith In Solutions / Resolution

I believe we should make reasonable attempts to validate the patient's faith in their future. This means that when they say they wouldn't kill themselves because their old girl friend wants them back we should attempt to speak with the girlfriend. It is not always reasonable to attempt to validate their hopes and plans for the future but you should make a reasonable attempt.

In some cases their idea of the future may be delusional or nearly delusional such as God telling them that they are going to win the lottery. Attempt to determine how they will react if this delusional hope does not materialize.

2. Indifferent / Ambivalent

This patient gives us very little to go on in either direction. They clearly have no reason to be optimistic but they also don't seem to be driven towards suicide either. I generally ask them if there is something that would give them hope, or if there is something that could cause them to take their life.

3. No Hope

This may occur in the midst of significant changes in life such as the death of a loved one or the loss of a relationship. It may also occur in the midst of depression. In either case an inpatient stay should be considered.

Notes:

Demographic Risk Factors

An awareness of demographics is more a legal issue than a clinical one. It can be helpful to demonstrate that you considered the elevated risk but this information will never tell who is going to take their life or who is going to be safe.

I. Male

Men are 4 times likely than women to take their life but women are 6 times more likely to attempt suicide. This means that we will interview far less men than women. In my opinion when we interview a male patient we must be very careful to adjust our interview style. Many men have a lethal intolerance to ego injury. This is significant in two ways. The first is the potential ego injury that may have precipitated the suicide interview. The second is the ego injury of the interview itself, it may be difficult for men to ask for help. Men in general will be more guarded.

In the event that the patient has suffered a loss, primarily a relationship loss but any loss to include a job, we need to determine if they have the coping skills to absorb the loss and move towards healing. In some cases the patient needs time to come to terms with the loss as they develop a broader perspective of the situation.

II. Lives Alone / Widowed / Separated

The highest risk population is widowed Caucasian elderly males. They may need some time to adjust to the loss of their spouse and gain some sense of purpose and a continued will to live. This may require a brief hospitalization.

III. Native American

This population represents higher risk for a variety of reasons that are as diverse as the geographic locations Native American people live in. One of the significant risk factors is related to a deep sense of spirituality many Native Americans have. This spirituality may remove some of the fear of death as it is viewed simply as one more step in a long journey. In addition, alcohol abuse and a history of sexual abuse may play a significant role.

IV. Family history of suicide

It is important to ask the patient their thoughts about family member suicides. In some cases the patient feels that suicide is "endorsed" as a viable option. In other cases they will say the family member suicide is why they would never take their life because they saw the pain it caused others. Be aware of "anniversary effect" related to family suicides. The anniversary can be the actual date of the suicide or the age of the individual who took their life. Clearly this anniversary can be a critical event for the patient.

V. Self harm

Self harm is a very important issue in suicide assessment. Of critical importance is how you document this section. You need to use the patient's words and indicate why they injured themselves such as; "I cut to relieve tension, express anger, feel alive, etc." In addition, document their own words regarding their thoughts about suicide such as; "I wasn't trying to kill myself, I would never kill myself that way." The average jury member will assume that all acts of self harm, especially wrist cutting are suicide attempts. You need to clearly address the issue of suicidal ideation or lack of ideation.

I address self harm within to the concept of alexithymia. Alexithymic patients cannot assign words to their emotions. In addition, they cannot share their emotions with others. This proves to be a significant problem as we are all somewhat compelled to share outlying emotional states both good and bad. Pain hurts less when we share it with others and joy is richer when shared as well.

Clearly visible self mutilation tends to simply be a "see my pain" statement. This most often occurs on the wrists and forearms. These patients appear less likely to engage in truly suicidal behavior as the intent of their action is to involve others in their emotional state. This can be actually protective. The self mutilation that is more hidden is often of greater concern. These patients are not communicating with others, they appear to be sending a self destructive message to themselves. They deserve to suffer, they should be punished. This is often a sign of sexual abuse. This topic should be approached carefully. The assessment process is not the time to begin trauma work with an abused patient.

Child Suicide Assessment

The assessment of children for suicide risk can be very brief if the caregivers has concerns about the child. There is almost no situation where we would force a caregiver to take a child home from the emergency department when they feel the child is at risk for self harm. We always accommodate the wishes of reasonable parents and caregivers. Certainly this changes after multiple visits, or if the parents appear to be engaging in factitious disorder by proxy which is when a caregiver willing misrepresents someone under their care as having a mental illness.

On some occasions the caregiver is concerned about the child but does not have strong feelings regarding hospitalization. In this situation we should clearly error on the side of caution. If the child gives you anything but clear negative responses to your inquires regarding suicide you should consider hospitalization.

The four primary areas of concerns are (according to Dr. Robert E. Larzerele):

I. Out Of Home Placement.

Children who are removed from home frequently have been subjected to abuse and neglect. As most children are still egocentric they feel that they are responsible for both the abuse and the trouble their caregiver is in. These children require very special attention if they are to navigate this difficult chapter of their life.

II. Perceived Lack Of Social Support.

It is common for children to feel as if no one understands them or cares about them. This is sometimes referred to as "disposable child syndrome." We need to clearly ask them if anyone cares about them. We pay attention to their perception regarding this topic. It does little good to inform them that people care about them, they need to perceive care.

III. Worsening Depression.

In cases where a child does not seem to have a sense of optimism regarding their future I become very concerned. Children focus so much on the short term it is easy for them to get a sense of hopelessness. I do not count on my ability to change their outlook in one simple interview. If they appear to be hopeless I often hospitalize. Remember that a significant indicator of hopeless depression is sleep disturbances. I am especially concerned about insomnia versus hypersomnia.

IV. Comfort With Death.

Most children understand that death is permanent so I am not overly concerned that children may believe that they will come back after they die. I am concerned about their attitude regarding death. Do they believe they will get to be with a loved one who has recently died?

In situations where you feel there is risk but the parent does not, you need to consider if the risk is significant enough to merit legal action, or can the parent just be strongly encouraged to seek outpatient services? In cases where action is called for Child Protective Services must be contacted.

Method Of Child Suicide:

When children do take their life they most often choose hanging. I am not sure if this is because they see fewer options or if it is because they want a self punishing manner of death. Remember that children being egocentric blame themselves for every bad thing in their world. It makes sense that many children feel a need to punish themselves. Anytime a child tells me they are thinking of hanging as a manner of suicide I pay very close attention.

Adolescent Suicide Assessment

The assessment of adolescents for suicide risk should be conducted using the same format as adult risk assessment.

The clinician must specifically focus on impulsivity and access to means.

Generally, it is recommended that if an adolescent presents for an assessment the parent, or legal guardian, must be present at the hospital as well as give permission to the clinician prior to the interview. One example of when this would not be the case is if the child were a ward of the state. In which case, the case worker would need to provide permission for the clinician to perform the risk assessment. This is also true for children.

The current standard of care is to hospitalize the adolescent unless there is a compelling reason to discharge them to a less restrictive level of care. Keep in mind that a parent has the right to decline admission to care.

If, in the clinician's judgement, the parent is acting in good faith and has the ability to ensure his or her child's safety a discharge could be in order. Prior to discharge the clinician should attempt to offer follow-up appointments with area providers, ensure means restriction by removing potential items to be used in suicide, as well as WARN the parent about the consequences of failing to follow the recommendations. It is also crucial to document this conversation as well as have the patient and parent sign and date a Safety Plan.

In the case where the clinician feels that the child or adolescent needs a higher level of care and therefore you disagree with the parent or guardian contact with Child and Family Services will be necessary.

A referral for medical neglect can result in this agency opening a case and monitoring the situation. In some cases, such as imminent suicide risk or severe and chronic mental illness, parents have temporarily lost their custodial rights due to their failure to act in their child's best interest.

Many times the threat of a medical neglect report is enough to spur the parent or guardian to consent to a higher level of care for their child.

Suicide Risk Potential

I. No Elevation.

This is the best we can ever say. There is no elevated risk. We never say "no risk".

Everyone has suicide risk but not everyone has elevated suicide risk. This conclusion has two parts, yours and the patient's. You see no indicators of suicide such as the presence of a mental illness and the patient denies current suicidal ideation or intent.

II. Mild

This patient has indicators of suicide such as depression or posttraumatic stress disorder but they deny suicidal ideation or intent.

III. Moderate

This patient has both the indicators of suicide such as a mental illness and suicidal ideation but they deny intent. In addition we must conclude that their denial was made in "good faith". We don't simply parrot what the patient says; we make an evaluative judgment of the patient's statements.

IV. High

Strong ideation with intent.

This is an easy conclusion to arrive at as the patient has indicators of suicide as well as suicidal ideation and intent. Hospitalization is the obvious choice here.

Disposition Based Upon Risk Potential

The goal of risk assessment is to determine if the patient represents a level of risk that requires inpatient treatment, or if the level of risk is acceptable enough to allow the patient to pursue outpatient options.

The manner in which we document this finding is often a subject of discussion amongst risk assessment professionals. One school of thought believes that if you keep your record sparse there is less for an attorney to attack in the event of a bad outcome. This always strikes me as somewhat naive because it assumes that we will not be held accountable for the substance of our assessment, we will just be held accountable for what we wrote about our assessment. In the real world we will be held accountable for both, the assessment and what we wrote about the assessment.

I believe the best compromise is this. We conduct a rich assessment demonstrating that we have considered a range of mental illnesses that the patient may be suffering from. We consider how these potential mental illnesses may combine with the current risk factors which include patient statements and actions as well the statements and actions collateral sources have attributed to the patient. We consider the patient's history and statements about intended course of actions. We then determine if the risk present requires inpatient or out patient treatment.

It may not be best to indicate what level of risk the patient represents such as low, medium or high risk, it may be best to simply indicate if the level or risk can be treated in an in-patient or out-patient setting.

Deterrents To Suicide

I. Loved Ones

Living with blood relatives is generally considered to be the strongest protective factor in the prevention of suicide. Close family ties clearly help distressed individuals cope with loss and change.

II. Spiritual Faith

People of faith do kill themselves less but data is conflicting on how much less. In part it depends on where the patient lives. People in the Bible belt tend to fear Hell as a punishment for suicide more than people who live in California. One theory states that people of faith are affiliated with other people of faith and that affiliation provides a protective buffer in the patient's life.

III. Hope For The Future

I frequently ask patients what they believe their future holds; I always ask this of inmates in jail settings. People with a reason to live and an optimistic outlook are less likely to take their life.

IV. Other

Sometimes I rather bluntly ask "Why wouldn't you take your life?" I do this in cases where I am having a difficult time reading the patient. It tends to catch the guarded patient a bit off guard; they may be more likely to give an honest response. Patients who are conflicted regarding their intentions may need to be confronted with harsh the reality of ending their life. This may force them to define a reason for living.

Specific Risk Inquiry: Violence or Homicide

Introduction:

Mental illness is not an independent predictor of violence. We are looking for mental illness in concert with the following: A history of violence, stated intent to commit a violent act and an egosyntonic relationship with violence. These three elements when combined with a mental illness represent significant risk.

It is important to note that mental illness does not make a person become violent; it may reveal violence in those who have the temperament for aggression. Mental illness may loosen ones grip on violent behavior making them much more likely to commit a violent act. This violence is most often in the presence of perceived or possibly actual provocation. At real issue here is perceived provocation. Many individuals with psychotic illnesses have a very difficult time reading non-verbal cues and may mistake normal social behavior as hostile.

When you encounter a patient who appears to be suffering from persecutory or paranoid thoughts it is important to ask them "What might you have to do to protect yourself?" I generally follow that question with "Do you think you could ever hurt someone before they hurt you?'

I. Has Physically Attacked Someone

As with nearly all human behavior, the past is the best predictor of the future when considering the risk of impending violence. Previous violence against others is clearly our best indicator of a patient's likelihood of future violence. It is very important to understand what provocation may have been present or perceived as present. We need to assess the likelihood that they will encounter this situation again. In addition, if their violent behavior had to be stopped by a third party you can infer that their behavioral goals went beyond self defense and may represent true aggression.

II. Reportedly Has Threatened To Harm Someone

This is typically why you are conducting the interview. First we attempt to determine if the report is credible. It is very important to talk to everyone involved, this includes the individual who claims to have heard the report first hand, the dispatcher who likely received the report and the officer who initially responded to the call. I generally do not interview the patient until I have spoken with all of the collateral sources.

Has threatened to harm someone in the presence of this interviewer. If the patient is making statements that suggest self defense is the motive for the threatened violence we then want to determine if the perceived threat is likely to be real or does it seem to be part of a delusion. In the event of a delusion you need to consider warning the potential victim. Keep in mind that not all states support the Tarasoff ruling issued in California.

Threats of harm that are not related to the perceived or actual need for self defense, and do not appear to be part of a delusional system may represent a crime and should be referred to law enforcement.

III. Entertains Thoughts Of Violence

Thoughts of violence are going to fall within three broad categories: self-defense, psychotic, criminal. We are clearly expected to address thoughts of violence that are related to psychosis, which can be defined as greatly impaired reality testing. Violence motivated by self-defense can also be the result of impaired reality testing. Criminal violence needs to be addressed by law enforcement and is outside of our scope of practice.

IV. Has Access To Means/Weapons

As a rule we are expected to make an effort to have weapons removed from the home of individuals who may be at risk for violence related to a mental illness. This can be difficult, as we have no legal grounds to do so in most cases. Generally we ask a family member to remove and keep the weapons for a time. Ideally we would reassess the patient before the weapons are returned but this is rarely done.

V. Has Taken Steps To Secure Means

A patient who has recently acquired a weapon should be viewed as a high risk.

VI. Reports Command Hallucinations

Patients with command hallucinations related to suicide are also high risk. It is crucial to determine if this represents a chronic state or is this something new. In the case of new auditory symptoms it may be best to evaluate and manage this patient in an inpatient environment. If their symptoms are chronic attempt to determine if the patient will be able to continue to resist the commands.

VII. Reckless Use Of A Weapon

This patient has very high risk of interpersonal violence, like the patient who habitually engages in the destruction of property, they are egosyntonic with violence and are willing to use violence to achieve their goals.

VIII. Destruction Of Property

The issue here is the apparent egosyntonic relationship with violence along with the use of violence as either emotional regulation or goal acquisition. These patients are at high risk for interpersonal violence.

Risk Of Adolescent Violence

I. Leakage

One of the most important factors in the assessment of violence in students is the concept of leakage. Leakage is the intentional or unintentional revelation of clues to feelings, thoughts, attitudes and possible actions. It may reflect an inner conflict that the student cannot resolve alone. It may be an actual cry for help or it may be boasting prior to committing a violent act.

The FBI has developed a protocol for the assessment of threats made in school settings.

www.fbi.gov/publications/school/school2.pdf

II. Nature Of The Threat

The first step is to determine the type of threat. Is it a **direct threat** such as "I am going to blow this school up." Is it an **indirect threat** such as "if I wanted to I could blow this school up." Veiled threats are even weaker such as, "my life would be better if I blew this school up." Or they may make a conditioned threat such as "I am going to blow this school up if they don't let me leave the campus for lunch." As a rule direct threats will always carry the most weight but no threat can be ignored.

Factors that should be considered include plausible details that indicate thought and planning. A student who states "I am going to kill Mr. Smith" is clearly making a threat but compare that to a student who says "I am going to shoot Mr. Smith Saturday morning when he takes his dog to the park to play fetch." The second student's statement indicates planning and preparation.

Implausible details imply less likelihood of actual violence. A student who threatens to "blow up every teachers car" is less likely to act than the student who threatens to light the principles car on fire.

III. Emotional Content Of The Threat

It may surprise you to learn that the degree of emotion associated with a threat has no correlation to acting on the threat.

IV. Personality Factors Associated With Violent Students

A. Absence Of Coping Skills

Students who lack coping skills have no way to defend themselves from unpleasant experiences with others. This may lead to the "kindling effect" where small offenses combine until the student feels overwhelmed by the weight of them all and feels they must act.

B. Expression Of Affect

Students who demonstrated emotional distress on either end of the spectrum may be at risk for violence. Rage or sadness may be a motivator. A sense of humiliation can be an extremely strong motivator for suicidal or homicidal behavior.

C. Lack Of Resilience

Students who seem to lack the ability to "bounce back" after disheartening experiences may be at risk for violence. This requires someone who has a longitudinal perspective of the student's life as well as the recent events in the students life.

D. Response To Authority

Either passive aggression or overt aggression to authority may be an indicator of potential violence.

E. A Sense Of Rejection

Rejection can be one of the most painful emotions we feel. In the case of a failed relationship males are 4 times more likely to take their life than females. When someone feels rejected by a peer group the risk of violence to others increases.

F. A "Hit" List.

Many teens will construct a "hit list" in response to feeling bullied or humiliated. In most cases they do not act on the list. It is important to ask a student if they have a list, how long they have had the list and if they believe they will actually act on the list.

G. Evidence Of A Strong Need For Control

Students with narcissistic features need to feel in control of everyone and everything around them. These students will often harbor ill feelings for a long time and may experience increasing rage and a need to retaliate.

H. Intolerance Of Others

Intolerance in any form such as religion, race, faith or sexual orientation can provoke a student to violent action. As a rule their intolerance is known as they find it difficult to hide their strong emotions.

I. Paranoia

Paranoia in children and adolescents is often less related to psychosis and more related to being raised by paranoid parents who speak of distrust of authority or certain groups of people. In the case of apparent psychosis the student should always be evaluated in an inpatient setting. In the case of deep distrust the student should be asked if they feel they will need to initiate a violent act to protect themselves. They will almost always make a point of saying that they will defend themselves if needed, this is not our primary concern, we want to know if they feel the need to be proactive regarding violence.

J. Fascination With Violence

Do they demonstrate in increasing fascination with violence? Are they watching violent movies or playing violent video games with increasing frequency? There is not yet solid research linking violent video games and movies with acts of violence but there is research to suggest that an increasing preoccupation with violence is an indicator of future violence. It is likely that violent video games and movies will never be linked to violent behavior because there is no ethical way to force a control group of children to watch violent movies or play violent games.

K. Fascination With Violent Role Models

Asking a student who they admire in history can be very revealing if the student identifies with a violent person such as Hitler.

L. Lack Of Empathy

The new diagnostic criteria for Conduct Disorder includes individuals who are callused and unemotional. These students demonstrate no remorse when they harm someone physically or emotionally.

M. Dehumanizing Language Or Actions

Students who speak of others in degrading terms or who seem to view others as objects are more likely to engage in violent acts towards others.

N. Demonstrations Of Inferiority

Students who make efforts to improve social status but are unsuccessful may engage in acts of violence.

O. Appearing Alienated

Students who speak of feeling alienated from others or who appear to be emotionally and physically isolated from others may engage in acts of violence.

P. Depression

Depression is clearly a risk factor for suicide but may also be associated with violence towards others.

Q. Family Dynamics Related To Violence.

Students who commit acts of violence tend to come from turbulent homes. These homes tend to lack structure and the children have not learned to responds to limits. Violence in the home is also a strong predictor of violent behavior.

R. School Factors That Increase Likelihood Of Violence.

Schools that tolerate bullying and allow the development of a "caste system" are more likely to have violent acts committed.

Risk Of Elderly Violence

With an increasing population of elderly, expect to see an increase in risk assessments of patients with dementia as well as behavioral disturbances. Assessing risk in the elderly population mainly centers on risks of danger to self or others or an inability to meet or care for their own needs.

> When assessing risk for elderly individuals consider that elderly white males above the age of 85 have the highest suicide rate compared to any other age or ethnicity.

Frequently, this patient will have been placed at a nursing home or partial care facility and will come to the attention of the mental health clinician after the patient assaults or attempts to assault one of the nurses or nurse's aids.

In the case of an aggressive elderly patient, it is generally necessary to place this person on an emergency detention or involuntary hold as they are not capable of making an informed consent to voluntarily enter a treatment facility. *Check with your county attorney's office for exact details on this issue.*

The grounds for the detention will generally be an imminent risk of danger to self or others as evidenced by the patient harming or attempting to harm others. By conducting a thorough examination of documentation and by interviewing the patient and the caregivers, a case can be established regarding the patient's history of aggression or violence. Generally, most nursing facilities give these patients numerous chances and finally something has to be done.

A second case for involuntary admission can be made by considering that the patient is unable to meet or care for their own needs. Frequently the patient is unable or unwilling to perform such tasks as eating, bathing, or even moving. In this situation it is crucial to consider this patient's functioning prior to the current behavioral disturbance as well as rule out possible medical issues which may have exacerbated the current condition.

It is interesting to note that urinary tract infections can have a significant effect on a patient's behavior as well as mental health condition.

Collateral Information

The need for collateral information cannot be overstated in high risk situations where the patient has previously made suicidal statements or has attempted suicide. In these situations I insist that the patient provide me with a collateral source, preferably a family member or spouse. If they refuse I generally tell them that I cannot effectively conduct a risk assessment so I will have to **involuntarily** admit them to the psychiatric unit for further assessment.

In most crisis situations the issue of confidentiality is not of concern. However, when the patient does provide me with a collateral source I generally ask the patient to first speak with the person and explain the situation we are in. This is true for both phone contact and face to face contacts when the collateral source is present at the Emergency Room.

My purpose in doing this is twofold. I first want to gauge the nature of their relationship; second, it avoids the issue of confidentiality as I have not given the collateral source any information, the patient has. I make it a practice to rarely if ever provide information to collateral sources, I get information from them rather than allow them to get information from me.

Again, issue of confidentiality is in many cases moot when managing psychiatric emergencies but I rarely break confidence even when it is legal for me to do so. If the patient will not willingly allow me access to collateral sources and will not willingly participate in the interview process I am very unlikely to allow them to leave under any condition. The collateral interview is unnecessary when I am interviewing an uncooperative patient; their refusal to enter into a good faith interview pre-determines the inpatient disposition by default.

When law enforcement is involved I always make an effort to speak directly with the responding officers and the officer who transported the patient from the scene to the ER. In addition, I attempt to speak with the dispatcher who received the original call. In the event the patient was transported via ambulance it is important to speak with the ambulance attendant. The information I receive from these individuals has been pivotal on many cases.

Collateral information should be gathered from family members as well as other individuals that are involved in your patient's life.

Consider contacting the resources listed below for additional collateral information.

Professional Contacts

A therapist or treatment provider can prove to be a crucial contact in establishing safety for a patient who is being released.

It is important to document the nature of their relationship, length of time they have been seeing the patient as well as a statement on their opinion of the patient's risk level.

Medical / Law Enforcement

This group includes the first responders (whether it is ambulance or law enforcement), as well as the dispatch operator who took the initial call.

It can also include the triage nurse at the medical facility, the direct care nurses and the emergency room physician.

Community Contacts

Neighbors can also provide important collateral contact information if they have an established relationship with the patient. They can provide insight into how this patient is functioning in society.

PART THREE

Disposition

The entire interview is intended to resource you to make an informed decision based on the best available information and your clinical insight. This is not the time for your "gut feeling" or intuition. In the event of a bad outcome it will be clear that your intuition was wrong. Your disposition must be supported by definable and professionally accepted standards of assessment. Keep in mind that malpractice is not outcome dependent, it is process dependant. The outcome is not on trial, your process of assessment is.

As I have stated previously, I am a believer in "defensive assessments". As you formulate your decision you must imagine doing so in a court room responding to a hostile attorney who is determined to present you as lazy, incompetent or both. This is not the time for shortcuts.

Your Disposition Must Be Supported By The Following Elements.

1. Clinical interview to determine the presence of a mental illness.

2. Contact with all collateral sources with attention paid to the reconciliation of possible discrepancies in their version and the patient's.

3. An awareness of the patient's history of dangerous behavior to self or others.

4. An awareness of the patient's history of compliance or non-compliance with previous treatment and or interventions.

5. The patient's willingness and ability to participate in a crisis and or treatment plan.

Two Paths Of Case Disposition

Patient Disposition

Clinical Disorders

The general rule for risk is the clinician bears the responsibility to manage the risk.

These patients are generally considered to be suffering from a serious and debilitating mental illness; as such they cannot be expected to manage their own mental health needs.

Clear indications for admission include psychosis, stated suicide intent or an inability to maintain personal safety. In some cases patients demonstrate an inability to meet or care for their own basic needs.

Personality Disorders

The general rule regarding risk is that the clinician is responsible to resource the patient to manage their own risk.

Risk in this presentation is chronic and therefore cannot be treated in an inpatient setting.

At times an acute, identifiable stressor will be present. In these cases, when there is a treatable goal, an inpatient stay may be advisable

Disposition Based Upon Risk Potential

The goal of risk assessment is to determine if the patient represents a level of risk that requires inpatient treatment, or if the level of risk is acceptable enough to allow the patient to pursue outpatient options.

The manner in which we document this finding is often a subject of discussion amongst risk assessment professionals. One school of thought believes that if you keep your record sparse there is less for an attorney to attack in the event of a bad outcome. This always strikes me as somewhat naive because it assumes that we will not be held accountable for the substance of our assessment, we will just be held accountable for what we wrote about our assessment. In the real world we will be held accountable for both, the assessment and what we wrote about the assessment.

I believe the best compromise is this. We conduct a rich assessment demonstrating that we have considered a range of mental illnesses that the patient may be suffering from. We consider how these potential mental illnesses may combine with the current risk factors which include patient statements and actions as well the statements and actions collateral sources have attributed to the patient. We consider the patient's history and statements about intended course of actions. We then determine if the risk present requires inpatient or out patient treatment.

It may not be best to indicate what level of risk the patient represents such as low, medium or high risk, it may be best to simply indicate if the level or risk can be treated in an in-patient or out-patient setting.

> ## Voluntary Admission:
>
> A psychiatrist accepts the patient based on the identification of acute stressors or mental illness that represents danger to self or others.
>
> These patients must be able to make a "*voluntary good faith statement*" regarding their desire for treatment. Intoxicated or psychotic patients cannot make voluntary good faith statements and should not be admitted under voluntary status.
>
> I recommend assessing intoxicated patients for risk after the Blood Alcohol Level is below 0.100.

Inpatient Disposition

There are two paths for inpatient disposition. Voluntary admission provides for the patient who is able to make a "voluntary good faith statement" and involuntary admissions or mental health holds apply to patients who are clearly at risk and in need of inpatient treatment are unable to or unwilling to consent to inpatient treatment.

The admitting psychiatrist will generally want to review the case prior to accepting a voluntary admission. This includes reviewing the circumstances leading to the risk assessment, the results of your risk assessment, as well as information that you have gathered from collateral contacts.

It will also be necessary to provide a provisional diagnoses as well as review the patient's current medications. If there are medical concerns it is important to ask the emergency room physician to review these concerns with the admitting psychiatrist prior to inpatient admission.

If this patient is elderly or has a medical condition that requires skilled care the treatment facility will also need to know that the patient is ambulatory and able to perform his or her own self-care such as feeding and hygiene. Prior to admission the inpatient nursing staff may perform a nursing assessment to ensure that they can meet the patient's needs.

The psychiatrist may also want to review the lab work as well as medical work-up prior to accepting the admission. Unless you have an established relationship with the admitting psychiatrist or the treatment facility it may be necessary to complete voluntary admission forms prior to acceptance of the patient for admission.

> ## Involuntary Admission:
>
> This patient must have a mental illness that clearly causes the patient to be at risk of causing harm to self or others. This is occasionally referred to as D.T.S. and D.T.O.; Danger to self or danger to others. In addition, the danger has to appear to be "imminent."

Every State will have their own specific wording for mental health hold but in general every state will require the clinician to demonstrate two things; the presence of a serious mental illness and the presence of imminent risk. The latter is considerably more difficult than the former.

Identification of a serious mental illness is as simple as listing the defining criteria for the mental illness, such as Schizophrenia or Major Depression. Establishing imminent risk is subjective and therefore open to interpretation.

Rarely will you find "imminent" defined. Like most laws, the intent is to allow latitude in interpretation. I always define imminent risk as action that is likely to occur within the next 24 hours. As evidence I can generally only offer two things, the patient's own statements and actions. In some cases we can use past acts to establish risk. Occasionally you may attempt to commit a patient based on things friends and family claim they have

> ### Imminent Risk:
>
> Action that is likely to occur within the next 24 hours

said. This is rarely successful. In the event that this case makes it into court the hearsay statue will prevent you from repeating these alleged statements. Friends and family will be required to testify in person and may be reluctant to do so.

As a general rule civil commitments are reserved for psychotic patients. These patients can benefit from involuntary treatment because they can be given anti-psychotic medications via injection. In time, the medication should mediate the risk. Patients who cannot be treated with medication are less frequently committed as they are far less likely to benefit from involuntary treatment.

The admitting psychiatrist will also need to know the same information regarding medical testing and examination as you would provide for the voluntary admission.

Transferring To Inpatient Treatment

There are a number of issues to carefully consider when transferring a patient to inpatient treatment. Transferring from one location to another should only be done by ambulance or by law enforcement.

This patient has undergone a complete medical assessment as well as a risk assessment. It is currently known what substances are in the patient's system. You should also know that the patient does not have any means of harming themselves or others. Do not allow this patient to have access to means after they are medically cleared. They may try to exit the moving vehicle.

Consider the safety of the patient and the community. Secure transportation is crucial if this patient is suicidal or homicidal. Do not allow this patient to be transferred in a personal vehicle for the same reasons listed above.

Do not consider transferring any patients to inpatient treatment in your own personal vehicle. This is a great risk and liability issue.

Outpatient Disposition

The heart of the outpatient disposition is the Crisis Agreement or Safety Plan. The issue here is one of "informed consent."

I. The No Self Harm Contract

These contracts have no legal value and should not be used. They may have some clinical value, particularly with patients who feel they have a strong therapeutic alliance with the clinician. A "crisis agreement" or "safety plan" should be used rather than the traditional "contract."

II. The Crisis Agreement or Safety Plan

Here are the components of a crisis agreement or safety plan.

- Does the patient have the ability to make an informed decision regarding their care and their best interest?
- Has the patient been informed of all treatment options including inpatient and outpatient and the benefits of each option?
- Have they been given a "good faith opportunity" to choose the option that best suits their needs?
- Do you agree that their choice adequately addresses their risk factors?
- Have they assured you that they both know how, and are willing to increase their level of care (i.e. crisis line, hospital, 911) if they are feeling unsafe or overwhelmed?
- Has the patient identified a person that is willing to monitor them after discharge? Have you, as the clinician, spoken to this person and alerted them of the circumstance of the situation, as well as what is needed?
- Is the identified person capable of supporting the patient?
- Have you adequately addressed means restriction?
- Is the patient willing to follow-up with a mental health care professional the following day as well as contact you as the risk assessment professional to check in regarding safety?
- Does the patient have a scheduled appointment with a mental health care provider? If so, identify the person, time and date.
- Seek a release of information to provide risk assessment information regarding to their care providers

Means Restriction

There is an old story in suicide literature called the British Coal Gas Story. It can be found in the British Journal of Preventative and Social Medicine (June 1976, P. 85).

This story is about a significant reduction in suicide rates that correspond with change from Coal Gas which is highly lethal and Natural Gas which is significantly less lethal. The number of suicides by gas dropped significantly and that drop was reflected in a drop in the total number of suicides. It appears that if an easy means of suicide were removed suicides diminished. Similar studies on bridge barriers have yielded similar results provided other bridges were not in close proximity.

This reduction in suicide strongly suggests that the time delay introduced via means restriction can have a lasting effect in suicide prevention. Many will say that if someone is going to kill themselves there is nothing anyone can do about it. This may be true for some, but for many the desire to die represents a very brief chapter in their lives. For some it may merely be a paragraph or even a sentence. If we can delay their ability to take their life it will give them time to turn a page and begin a new chapter. There is substantial value in means restriction.

Means Restriction:

The reduction of access to means—weapons, rope, poison, drugs, etc.—as well as risk reduction—e.g., detoxifying automobile exhaust or cooking gas—for suicide on the premise that fewer people would commit suicide if the means were not available.

Case Studies

Case Study #1: Intoxicated And Seeking Attention

Case Study #2: Homeless With Psychosis

Case Study #3: From Incarcerated To Inpatient

Case Study #4: Male With Persecutory Delusions

Case Study #5: Child With Behavioral Problems

Case Study #6: New Mom With Postpartum Depression

Case Study #7: Patient Says I Will Stab Myself.

Case Study #8: He Said She Said. (Version One)

Case Study #9: He Said She Said. (Version Two)

The case studies are composites of situations that could occur during mental health risk assessments.

They do not depict any one case or even any ten cases. The names used in the case studies are not intended to imply that the person or persons were actually involved in these events.

Case Study #1: Intoxicated And Seeking Attention

<u>Presenting Problem</u>

A family member contacted "911" after she learned that her son, Tommy, had "slit his wrist with a razor and was suicidal." Dispatch sent out an "attempt to locate" on a 23-year-old male who was last seen walking along a busy roadway. Tommy was located by law enforcement. The patient was transported to the emergency department for medical treatment as well as a mental health risk assessment.

Custody of the patient was given to hospital security due to the patient being on a "mental health hold." They remained at bedside and perform the necessary security protocol. Tommy was argumentative and caustic, stating that he had "done nothing wrong", "was being held against his will," and refused medical assessment. Tommy acquiesced after some time to examination by the emergency room physician. He refused to allow lab work.

Examination of the self-inflicted wounds on left forearm revealed superficial scrapes that did not require sutures. After completing the necessary medical evaluation and gaining more clarity into the gravity of this situation Tommy agreed to be cooperative. Security staff was asked to stand by and the patient agreed to allow the blood draw. His Blood Alcohol Level upon arrival was 0.225. The patient understood that he would need to stay at the emergency department until his Blood Alcohol Level was under 0.100 and the on-call mental health clinician could perform a risk assessment.

After Tommy was medically cleared and ready for discharge or transfer the mental health clinician was notified. He arrived and gained the following information through his mental health risk assessment. The self-inflicted wound was an attempt to get his girlfriend, Sarah, to "pay more attention to him." It appears that he and his girlfriend have worked things out and Sarah was present during the assessment. The mental health clinician also interviewed his mother, Kathryn, via telephone after securing the patient's permission to speak to her. (The clinician did not need the patient's permission in this situation but it is best to attempt to gain the patient's permission rather than appear to go behind the patient's back.

It also helps the patient know that his family is aware of the situation and can aide in discharge planning.)

Tommy's mood was stable and he believed his actions last night were "stupid." He admitted to drinking a fifth of whiskey, which resulted in reducing his inhibitions. Tommy does not believe that he intended to kill himself and adamantly denies wanting to harm himself today. He denies previous suicidal attempts or suicidal ideation. Mother and girlfriend also endorse this opinion as well.

Tommy believes that people who commit suicide take the "foolish way out ---- there's always help". He minimized past self-deprecating thoughts while intoxicated, which was reported by his girlfriend during interview with the mental health clinician.

Treatment History

Tommy has had no previous mental health treatment and has attended a court-ordered DUI class after his first charge 23 months ago. He has never attended AA or had intensive outpatient treatment for chemical dependency.

He denies previous suicidal ideation or attempts.

Disposition

Emergency room physician and on-call psychiatrist were consulted regarding discharging this patient to his mother's care.

Tommy was offered voluntary admission to the local psychiatric faculty but does not wish to go voluntarily and believes he can maintain his safety at home. His mother and girlfriend are in agreement with him regarding the Safety Plan. Tommy does not meet criteria for an emergency detention at this time.

Family denies presence of firearms in the house. Tommy denies having a plan to harm himself and identified his continued alcohol use as the primary stressor in his life. He recognizes that alcohol reduces inhibitions and he responds impulsively.

Tommy agrees to go to AA, agrees to follow up with the local chemical dependency center to address his chemical dependency issues. He was given a list of referrals to include the 24-hour mental health crisis line, AA meeting times, and a phone number for the local chemical dependency treatment center. His family was also provided copies of the referral information. Kathryn and Sarah voice understanding of what to do if the patient becomes a danger to himself or others. Tommy was warned and advised of the risks of not following up with the above plan as well as the possible negative consequences of continuing to abuse alcohol.

<u>This patient was discharged after considering the following information:</u>

- No previous suicide attempts
- Family and relationship support
- Family agrees with patient safety
- Patient has insight and deterrent in place
- Patient is amenable to outpatient treatment

===

Case Study #2: Homeless With Psychosis

<u>Presenting Problem</u>

Local law enforcement conducted a routine traffic stop on a vehicle with no left-turn signal. After approaching the vehicle they found Sharon, a 45-year-old female, with numerous driving violations and obviously in need of help. He called for assistance from a female officer who arrived a short time later. The vehicle plates indicated that the car was registered in a county about 135 miles to the north.

In addition to the broken turn signal, Sharon was driving with an expired driver's license and expired plates. The officer also observed that the windshield was severely damaged and there were no blades on the windshield wipers. He also observed that there was a dead cat in the front seat and another cat in the back appeared malnourished. Sharon's personal belongings and trash were piled to the ceiling obstructing views to safely operate the vehicle. There was cat feces throughout the car and the odor was overwhelming.

Sharon stated that she had just been kicked out of a homeless shelter yesterday, spent the night in her car, and was now headed to the airport to fly out of state for a "vacation." A yellow convertible passed and she yelled an expletive, flipped off the teenage boys in the car. Sharon told the officers that "they were the one's in on it getting Prissy (her cat) killed." During this time, her mood and behaviors vacillated between being angry and confused and from aggressive to total cooperation.

The officers correctly determined that Sharon was in need of mental health treatment and transported her to the local emergency department.

After arriving in the emergency department Sharon was observed responding to internal stimuli. Her speech is pressured and her mood was increasingly irritable. She believed that a dark-haired male nurse was also involved in her cat's death. Whenever she saw him Sharon became highly irritable and she was verbally aggressive. Her feet are dirty, she is unkempt, appears to have not showered recently.

Sharon was abrasive to other staff as well. She made various threats against the security officers who remain outside of her room due to the patient being on a "mental health hold." They perform the necessary security protocol after the patient is placed in hospital scrubs. Her belongings are searched for safety concerns, each item is carefully logged, and then stored in a locked cabinet until the patient is either released or transferred to another location. Law enforcement also was present during this time to provide support if needed. Sharon yells loudly at the officers and uses expletives, "* # @, you can't do this to me I am going on vacation." The law enforcement officers moved to a location in the department where they can respond if needed but will not further agitate the patient.

The emergency room physician attempted to perform a physical examination but Sharon was too agitated to allow her to do so. The physician offered Ativan to help the patient calm down. The patient initially refused but 10 minutes later she agreed after the charge nurse was able to encourage her cooperation. After 15 minutes, Sharon's agitation was sufficiently reduced and she was able to sit on her bed with less movement. She cooperated with the physical examination, allowed for a blood draw, and provided urine for analysis. She told the nurse that she was not taking any medication at this time. After reviewing the lab work the physician concluded that there were no medical complications and called the mental health clinician.

Upon arrival at the emergency department, the clinician reviewed the medical record and spoke to the law enforcement officers. Law enforcement had impounded her vehicle and disposed of the dead cat. The other cat was taken to the animal shelter where it will be cared for until Sharon is either discharged from treatment or a family member can pick the animal up.

The clinician also contacted the homeless shelter director to determine why Sharon was kicked out. The clinician learned that after 4 days at the shelter Sharon was asked to leave the homeless shelter due to her frequent intrusions into other resident's rooms. Sharon was also speaking loudly and yelling at the other residents. The homeless shelter director reported that the patient had discount coupons from a local grocery store that she believed were free airline tickets to an all-inclusive resort near Cancun, Mexico. The patient also was caring for her pets that she was keeping in her vehicle due to them not being allowed in the shelter. He also reported that the patient had eaten minimally and refused to regularly shower while in the shelter.

The clinician performed a risk assessment and found that Sharon was experiencing auditory hallucinations. Her speech was pressured, mood was irritable, thought processes are tangential, and she cited numerous delusions. When asked about her vacation plans Sharon changed the story and stated that the coupons were not "really" airline tickets they actually were valuable for banking and she planned to deposit them into her bank account. She estimated their value at $200,000. She was not able to explain what happened to her pets. Throughout this interview, the patient became more agitated when the clinician asked about her previous treatment history. Sharon ended the interview with the clinician on two occasions. During this time the clinician worked on her case notes and observed the patient responding to internal stimuli. Sharon told the clinician that she was talking to her cats.

The clinician asked Sharon if she could contact the patient's family members and she refused permission. In this case the clinician determined that the family's input, although helpful, would not substantially change the disposition of this case and used not calling the patient's family as a way to establish better therapeutic relationship with the patient.

Treatment History

The clinician was able to log on to the mental health center's secure database and learned that Sharon has an extensive history of serious mental illness.

Sharon has been enrolled at the mental health center for 52 months where she has received medication services, case management, and individual therapy. Her compliance to this program has been sporadic and her stability tenuous. Sharon has been prescribed an antipsychotic medication.

There have been four previous admissions to inpatient psychiatric facilities. Her first admission was 10 years ago in Nebraska where she spent 10 days in an inpatient mental health treatment center. She has also been to the local inpatient unit on 2 occasions and was committed to the state psychiatric hospital in South Dakota 3 years ago.

Disposition

Emergency room physician and on-call psychiatrist were consulted regarding detaining this patient on an emergency mental health hold. Sharon is not able to make a good faith voluntary admission and she is not stable enough to discharge back into the community.

Sharon clearly is unable to meet or care for her own needs and is also determined to be an imminent risk to self or others in the community. This is indicated by her aggressions towards others who she believes are responsible for her cat's death. She was given a copy of the emergency mental health hold paperwork as required by state law.

State law also requires the clinician to notify a family member of the emergency mental health hold. The patient's daughter, Mandy, was contacted and informed that her mother was placed at the inpatient psychiatric hospital on a hold as required by state law. Mandy was also provided contact information for the facility.

Sharon was transported to the inpatient psychiatric unit via ambulance and placed in the secure unit for observation and treatment. The clinician filed the paperwork with the county attorney's office in the patient's county of residence. The county attorney's office began the involuntary commitment process.

This patient was involuntarily admitted after considering the following information:

- Long-standing history of mental illness
- Previous inpatient psychiatric admission
- Clearly delusional
- Potential for danger to others
- Inadequate awareness of her surroundings
- Patient is not amenable to voluntary admission

Case Study #3: From Incarcerated To Inpatient

<u>Presenting Problem</u>

The mental health clinician is asked to assess a 38-year-old inmate, Robert, at the local detention center where he has been held for 21 days after violating a Restraining Order filed by his family. This violation was a misdemeanor.

Since his incarceration Robert has been receiving medications under the supervision of a psychiatrist who consults with the detention center and sees inmates every Wednesday. Robert has been taking Seroquel and Depakote. Robert had been on these medications in the past with good control over his positive symptoms of schizophrenia. Despite being on medications the inmate continued to exhibit psychotic behaviors and has continued to decompensate.

This morning Robert asked the detention officer who brought him breakfast if he liked the "Rembrandt" paintings on the cell walls that he made last night? The inmate was later observed washing carrot sticks in his toilet. Robert also flooded his cell and detention staff came in and cleaned it up.

The mental health clinician interviewed Robert who states he is not doing well and needs help. He readily volunteers information but when asked about the flooded cell he states, "I cleaned that up myself." Robert also tells the clinician that he has seen snakes crawling across his blanket. He has told the detention staff that he served with the Seabees in the Korean War as well as Operation Enduring Freedom. Robert also states that he has been a district court judge and he made an important decision to free a defendant in a high profile gun crime case in an adjoining state. When questioned about this Robert denied making these statements and states that he is really a "jack of all trades". He was been observed to be pacing and talking to himself in his cell.

The clinician concluded that the inmate is actively psychotic and his best interest is not being served by his current placement. Robert needs to be placed in a facility where his mental health needs can be more effectively addressed. The clinician contacted the judge who was willing to have the charges dropped and release this inmate providing that he be placed in an inpatient psychiatric facility.

The detention center supervisor arranged transport for this patient to the local emergency room for medical screening prior to admission to the inpatient psychiatric unit.

After arriving in the emergency department Robert is observed responding to internal stimuli. He is cooperative and grateful for the help offered. Robert tells the emergency room physician that he wants to go to the psychiatric hospital. He states that he was "scared and did not know what to do about the snakes" and that he was "exhausted from painting all night."

As per hospital protocol security officers remain outside of his room due to the patient being on a "mental health hold." He politely visits with them about the weather as well as his fishing trip to the mountains last summer. Robert willingly puts on hospital scrubs and agrees to be searched as well as the officers logging and placing his belongings in a locked cabinet until he is transferred to another location.

The physician offered Ativan and Haldol to help the patient calm down. The patient gratefully agreed to take the medications stating "I will do anything to get help to control the snakes." Robert cooperated with the physical examination, allowed for a blood draw, and provided urine for analysis. The physician concluded that there were no medical complications after reviewing the lab work.

The mental health clinician had already completed the necessary paperwork while at the detention center. He had also spoken to the on-call psychiatrist who agreed that the patient be placed on an emergency mental health hold pending results of the medical examination at the emergency department.

Treatment History

The clinician was able to log on to the mental health center's secure database and learned that Robert has an extensive history of serious mental illness.

Robert has been at the state psychiatric hospital on two occasions 3 and 6 years ago. He was released with a conditional release* on both occasions and managed to maintain stability when placed back in the community for about 18 months. It then appears that he begins to slowly decompensate and then begins to fail in treatment.

Robert engaged initially in services from the local mental health center and had been couch surfing with friends and family in the area. He has had numerous conflicts with his family and the crisis line receives calls frequently from his family.

<u>Disposition</u>

Emergency room physician and on-call psychiatrist were consulted regarding detaining this patient on an emergency mental health hold. Although this patient wants to go to the inpatient treatment facility he is deemed to not be competent at this time to make a good faith voluntary admission. He is not stable enough to discharge back to the detention center.

Robert clearly is unable to meet or care for his needs and is also determined to be an imminent risk to self or others in the community. He was given a copy of the emergency mental health hold paperwork as required by state law. State law also requires the clinician to notify a family member of the emergency mental health hold. The patient's sister, Janeen, was contacted and informed that her brother was placed at the inpatient psychiatric hospital on a hold as required by state law. The sister was also provided contact information for the facility.

The patient was transported to the inpatient psychiatric unit and placed in the secure unit for observation and treatment. The clinician filed the paperwork with the county attorney's office that began the involuntary commitment process.

<u>This patient was involuntarily admitted after considering the following information:</u>

Long-standing history of mental illness
Previous inpatient psychiatric admission
Clearly delusional
The psychiatrist agrees with the clinician that an involuntary hospitalization is the best course of action until the patient clears enough to make an informed decision regarding admission.

* Conditional Release:

A situation where a person is released from a state hospital prior to the completion of the court-ordered length of stay. In this situation certain conditions must be followed by the individual. If the conditions are violated the individual can be returned to the state hospital after a hearing to revoke the conditional release.

Case Study #4: Male With Persecutory Delusions

<u>Presenting Problem</u>

Martin came into the emergency department last night requesting admission to the local inpatient psychiatric facility because he felt that "his head was just not quite right." Prior to checking in to the emergency department he stated he needed to smoke a cigarette. He returned and rather than checking in slept most of the night in the waiting room. At 0430 Martin awoke, checked in, and again stated that he felt his "head was just not right." Hospital security staff was present and followed security protocol for patient safety.

The medical staff conducted the usual medical screenings and lab work and did not feel that there was any medical complication that could contribute to the patient's current complaint. The mental health clinician was called in to assist with disposition.

The clinician learned that Martin lives alone in an apartment near the downtown area of the city and is employed as a programmer for a large out-of-state software company. Martin works from his home office where he programs software for the banking industry. He states that his job performance has decreased and his boss has told him that he needs to "get things figured out or he will be let go." He began experiencing job performance difficulties about 6 months ago.

Martin has few friends and no extended family in the area. He was born and raised near Roswell, New Mexico and moved here 5 years ago because it was "not the desert." Martin denies the use of illicit drugs and alcohol. He smokes 1.5 packs of cigarettes each day. He also denied suicidal ideation or any previous suicide attempts.

After gathering background data as well as information related to previous mental health history, of which Martin had none, the patient asked the clinician if he believed someone could have "true ESP".

When asked for clarification Martin reported that in his opinion all of his difficulties are the result of Extra Sensory Perception. He feels that for the last 8 months "certain people" in town are preventing him from using his ESP; Martin also feels that "the local retailers have been selling him cigarettes laced with mind-controlling substances."

The clinician began to dig deeper into this delusion and became more concerned when Martin began to speak about two high profile women in town that he believes are specifically interfering with his ESP. One of them is a well-known realtor and the other is a prominent human rights activist. Martin states that the women have contacted law enforcement and now he is being investigated for child abuse. He does not know how they are controlling his mind but he is convinced that they have control over his life. Martin also said that the FBI and CIA are after him because they think he is abusing women.

Martin adamantly denied having any past history of violence yet there is a great deal of emotion around this topic of violence. It was not possible to determine if this patient has a history of assault or violence at this time.

The clinician was concerned about how his current delusions were influencing his behaviors and was especially concerned about the patient's potential to retaliate against the women whom he believes are falsely accusing him of child abuse or injure local cigarette retailers who he thinks might be involved in the plot to harm him.

Treatment History

There is no known record of previous treatment for this patient. He denies ever being on medication for mental illness.

Disposition

Martin appears to be suffering from persecutory delusions, which are likely due to paranoid schizophrenia. He was placed on an emergency mental health hold due to concerns about his potential for violence against women.

Emergency room physician and on-call psychiatrist were consulted regarding detaining this patient on an emergency mental health hold. Although Martin wants to go to the inpatient treatment facility he is deemed to not be competent at this time to make a good faith voluntary admission. Martin is not stable enough to discharge back to the community.

Martin was seen as an imminent risk to self or others in the community. He was given a copy of the emergency mental health hold paperwork as required by state law. State law also requires the clinician to notify a family member or other contact of the emergency mental health hold. The patient's friend, Sam, lives in Nevada, was contacted and informed that the patient was placed at the inpatient psychiatric hospital on a hold as required by state law. The friend was also provided contact information for the facility.

Martin was transported to the inpatient psychiatric unit via ambulance and placed in the secure unit for observation and treatment. The clinician filed the paperwork with the county attorney's office that began the involuntary commitment process.

<u>This patient was involuntarily admitted after considering the following information:</u>

- Clearly delusional
- Potential for danger to others with specific victims identified
- Inadequate awareness of his surroundings
- Patient is seeking voluntary admission but his behavior indicates that he will likely change his mind prior to arrival at the inpatient facility.

Case Study #5: Child With Behavioral Problems

<u>Presenting Problem</u>

This 8-year-old female, Chelsea, is brought to the emergency department for "mental health counseling" by her parents, Mike and Cindy, after she had her fifth anger outburst at school in the last month. She is crying and stating "I do not want to go in there."

Chelsea is triaged and placed in a hospital room pending medical assessment by the emergency room physician. The physician decided to not draw blood or conduct any other lab work after speaking to the parents. The physician charts in his notes that this case seems to be a behavioral problem and is not a crisis situation that requires risk assessment from the mental health clinician. The physician returns to the child's room and shares his opinion with the Mike and Cindy who become livid and insist that they want a mental health assessment and will not leave until their daughter is seen by the mental health clinician.

At a loss about what to do the emergency room physician calls the mental health clinician and asks for her assistance. The clinician informs the emergency room physician that she is at another hospital doing a risk assessment and it will be at least 45 minutes before she arrives for this assessment. The emergency room physician informs Mike and Cindy of this and they choose to wait.

After one hour and fifteen minutes the clinician arrives and meets Chelsea who now is sitting quietly on the bed eating a sandwich, crunching on potato chips, and drinking from a juice box. Mike and Cindy are present as well and are animated and obviously irritated that they had to wait so long for the clinician to arrive.

The clinician asks the parents to meet in the family support room so she can gain background information. The parents are well meaning but have little ability to parent this child. They treat her more like a peer rather than a child. The parents describe their daughter's behavior as pushing the limits at every opportunity. The daughter reacts strongly when told "no" or the parents attempt to redirect the child to a more acceptable behavior. Mike describes himself as stricter than his wife yet when asked for examples of setting appropriate limits he can provide none. Cindy describes herself as feeling guilty for having to place Chelsea in childcare after school and in the summers and wants to compensate for being away from her only daughter by letting her have and do what she wants. Cindy states that she does not like conflict.

After 45 minutes of interview time with the parents the clinician interviewed Chelsea who was enjoying playing with a rubber glove "balloon" provided by her nurse. Chelsea states that she does not know why she became angry at school but thinks that maybe her friends were being "mean" to her.

Treatment History

Chelsea has been seen by a local psychiatrist and has an established therapist at the local mental health center. She has been prescribed Resperidol in the past in hopes to moderate her mood swings. There has been little success in her treatment to change her behaviors.

Mike and Cindy also have an appointment scheduled with a child neurologist in a neighboring township.

Mike and Cindy have never participated in family counseling or attended any type of parenting classes despite the child's therapist recommending this as part of the treatment plan.

Disposition

The "identified patient" appears to be incorrectly identified. This is a parenting issue not a child behavioral problem.

At first, Mike and Cindy were insistent that their daughter be placed in the local inpatient psychiatric facility. Although there clearly is no reason to hospitalize this child the clinician decided to appease the parents by at least inquiring about inpatient treatment. The clinician contacted the admitting psychiatrist at the local psychiatric hospital where there is a policy against accepting children under the age of 13. She also contacted two out-of-town treatment facilities that actually accept children; they were full at this time. The parents then started to realize that they would need to take their daughter home.

The clinician carefully navigated this difficult situation by making observations about the behaviors Chelsea displayed at school, but especially at home. The clinician then broached the subject that perhaps Mike and Cindy could learn some other skills to help Chelsea learn to cope with the family dynamics. To help the parents learn these skills the clinician suggested that the parents enroll in parenting classes at the local family resource center and surprisingly they agreed to take the referral.

Overall, Mike and Cindy feel that they got some direction from the mental health clinician and they told her that they feel the time they spent at the emergency department was worthwhile.

<u>This patient was discharged after considering the following information:</u>

- Parents are legal guardians
- Parents are agreeable to outpatient counseling, which if they engage can likely address family issues
- Chelsea does not meet admission criteria
- Established relationship with outpatient psychiatrist

Case Study #6: New Mom With Postpartum Depression

<u>Presenting Problem</u>

A 26-year-old female, "Jenny", who is 6 week postpartum is seen at the OBGYN office with her newborn daughter for a well-baby check up. The physician examined the baby and found that everything with this newborn is great. When the physician asks Jenny how she is doing she begins to cry hysterically. She tells her doctor that she is having a difficult time and just does not feel good about being a mother. Jenny feels overwhelmed and out of touch with everything and everyone around her. Jenny stated that her mom left to return to her home about 10 days ago after being with them for 4 weeks. This is when she started to feel more depressed. Her husband, Todd, works shift work and is not around on a consistent basis.

The physician becomes more concerned when Jenny tells her that she has actually contemplated suicide and actually has a plan in place. Jenny states that she has acquired a large number of over-the-counter sleeping pills and she intends to ingest them with alcohol when Todd goes to work for his next night shift at the local lumber mill. Jenny sees no other way out of her depression and thinks she will always be a "terrible mother" to her baby. Jenny thinks that her daughter would be better off if she were dead and her daughter had a "different better" mother.

The physician spoke to Jenny about her concerns for safety as well as her need for treatment for her depression. Jenny agreed to speak to a mental health clinician and the doctor requested a risk assessment through the mental health crisis line at the mental health center. The doctor also called Todd who immediately came to the doctor's office from his work. He provided support to his wife, but previously had been unaware of his wife's depression or of her true intentions regarding suicide. Todd told the doctor that he thought his wife was just tired due to not getting enough sleep.

Before the mental health clinician arrived the couple had decided that they needed help to address Jenny's depression. They expressed concerns to the physician related to Jenny continuing to breast feed their daughter. The physician had ordered the necessary lab work and had her medical staff photocopy all of the pertinent medical records.

The mental health clinician performed the standard risk assessment with the intention of securing a voluntary admission to the inpatient psychiatric facility. Voluntary admission was given and Jenny went to the hospital for treatment.

Treatment History

There is no previous history of depression or mental health treatment. Although there is a past history of alcohol use there has been no use for the last 11 months.

Disposition

One of the biggest barriers to treatment for Jenny was the inability to breast-feed her baby. The clinician spoke to the inpatient treatment center staff to determine if it would be possible to either allow the child to breast feed at certain times of the day when the person caring for the baby could bring her in to nurse or if it is possible for Jenny to pump and have the milk stored for pick-up by the caregiver. The hospital was able to provide for both of these options.

Todd's parents live in the area and his mother was willing to provide childcare for her granddaughter while Todd was at work. They are also able to be involved in transporting their granddaughter to see her mom as well.

This admission is voluntary and the mental health clinician consulted with Jenny's physician as well as the on-call psychiatrist prior to receiving admission orders. In this case, all care providers agreed that Jenny could be transported to the inpatient unit by her husband in their personal vehicle*. Her husband was notified of the risks for failure to take his wife there as well as warned against stopping anywhere else prior to reaching the hospital.

After Todd sat with Jenny for the admission paperwork he and his daughter returned home and brought the breast pump, clothing, and personal care items to his wife at the inpatient unit.

<u>This patient was voluntarily admitted after</u>
<u>considering the following information:</u>

- Clearly depressed and in need of treatment
- Suicide plan in place with access to means
- Outpatient options cannot adequately ensured her safety
- Patient is seeking voluntary admission with support of her husband.

* Transportation To The Inpatient Facility:

Patients and their families will frequently ask if they can transport themselves to the inpatient unit rather than pay for an ambulance transfer. Most hospitals have an established policy regarding hospital transfers.

Generally, it is not wise to allow a patient to be transferred via private vehicle to an inpatient facility after the patient has entered the hospital or physician's office.

The clinician and admitting hospital need to be able to ensure that the patient does not have access to weapons, medications, or other means to harm themselves or others. They also need to be able to control the patient's access to illicit drugs or alcohol. They also need to prevent the potential for patient elopement.

Once the patient leaves the confines of a secured situation the potential for risk greatly elevates. This could potentially result in lawsuits for malpractice.

Case Study #7: Patient Says I Will Stab Myself.

<u>Presenting Problem</u>

Candice was brought to the local emergency department by friends after a night of drinking and then this morning reportedly stating, "I miss my boys, I'll stab myself." Last night, after an argument with her boyfriend, Brad, she drank two bottles of wine in five hours. When Candice awoke this morning she had severe stomach pains and made the self-harm statement. Brad dropped her off at the emergency department and left. He does not have a cell phone, it is his day off, and cannot be located.

Candice enters the emergency department voluntarily and agreed to all medical testing to address her stomach pain. After physical examination, Candice provided a urine specimen, and the phlebotomist drew blood. The samples were sent to the lab for processing. When the lab results were completed the emergency room physician reviewed the results and found to his surprise that Candice's Blood Alcohol Level was 0.230. The physician assumed that her Blood Alcohol Level was close to 0.080.

The emergency room staff informed Candice that they would need to re-draw the level in about 5 hours and she was in agreement to settle in and relax. In addition to a hospital breakfast tray, the physician ordered a "Banana Bag" to help replace fluids as well as speed the processing of the alcohol in her system. After the Blood Alcohol Level was under 0.100 the mental health clinician was called in to assess risk because of her self-harm statement. Candice also asked her nurse if she could call her sister-in-law, Sharon, who came to the hospital to sit with Candice.

The clinician conducts a risk assessment and observes that Candice is tearful and sad. Her chief complaint is "I miss my boys." Candice's two sons ages 4 and 6 live out of state about 3 hours drive from where she lives. She states that she really does not want to die, but sometimes her feelings of loss and no control are so great that she can see no alternate. This is especially true when she is drinking. She describes herself as a "binge drinker" and drinks 3 to 4 times per week. She repeatedly failed to maintain sobriety and this is why she chose to have her sons cared for by her brother and his wife. She has maintained all parental rights. Candice reports that she is unable to see the children due to the distance and she is working full-time. She feels that she cannot control when they will come home again.

Candice states that she has become more depressed over the last two years since her decision to place her sons with her brother. She reports sleeping 4 - 6 hours however wakes up immediately missing them. Candice does mention a 4 - month period of sobriety last year from September to December when she was able to contain the self harm thoughts. She denies any previous suicide attempts. She is actively involved working for a local landscape company and Candice is working about 40 to 50 hours per week. She states she eats well.

Candice was seen by a fellow mental health clinician three years ago for a similar presentation. The clinician recommended follow-up care at the local mental health center as well as the local chemical dependency center. Candice did not follow up on either of the referrals. She also has never had outpatient care or been on medications for depression.

Candice was offered the opportunity to make a voluntary admission to the inpatient treatment center and she declined at this time. She feels that she has a good support system she just did not use it. She states she would like to go to Sharon's house. The clinician informed Candice that inpatient treatment is an option for her if she feels she needs the extra support or if she is unable to feel safe once leaving the hospital. Candice also agrees to abstain from using alcohol for at least 48 hours. She also committed to attend her church's Celebrate Recovery program to help with her chemical dependency issues.

Candice's sister-in-law, Sharon, is present at the hospital and the clinician spoke to her to verify information. Sharon describes their family as "pretty close." Sharon is willing to stay with the client today and assist Candice getting to outpatient appointments from a chemical dependency evaluation as well to the medical appointment for consideration of starting an antidepressant medication. Sharon states that she is willing to have Candice stay "for as long as she needs to stay."

Candice began to attend a small local church about 4 months ago and appears to have a good relationship with the pastor's wife at the church as well as a number of ladies that are about her own age. Candice has been seeing the pastor's wife for "counseling" and she is willing to continue sessions with her. She is able to convincingly agree to a Safety Plan and stay away from alcohol.

Treatment History

Previous mental health risk assessment with Ruth Johnson from the local mental health center.

Referrals were provided and Candice did not follow through.

Disposition

Initially, the clinician had concluded that Candice needed to go to inpatient treatment for mental health treatment. She instead was able to determine that Candice has a good support system, no previous acts of self-harm, and is amenable to outpatient treatment. Case disposition was aided by the presence of Sharon and her willingness to take responsibility of her sister-in-law.

The Safety Plan covered all of the issues related to Candice's current needs and outlined the treatment recommendations as well as what steps were to be taken if Candice chose not to follow the Safety Plan. The clinician provided contact information for the various agencies that she referred Candice to as a way to prevent a barrier for accessing treatment. The hospital social worker also scheduled an appointment with Candice's medical provider for her follow-up for assessing if she needs to be prescribed an antidepressant. Chemical dependency treatment follow-up is most crucial at this time for Candice. She needs to be assessed and be seen by an outpatient chemical dependency counselor for treatment.

The clinician consulted with the emergency room physician and the on-call psychiatrist who agreed that Candice could be discharged to the care of Sharon provided that Candice agree to follow the Safety Plan.

The clinician also asked Candice to contact the crisis line the following day to "check-in" and report how she is doing.

This patient was discharged after considering the following information:

- Candice is in agreement for need of outpatient treatment
- Safety plan in place with adequate support
- Services are already in place.
- Patient agrees to abstain from alcohol.

Case Study #8: He Said She Said. (Version One)

<u>Presenting Problem</u>

Walker, a 36-year-old male, is brought to the emergency department by law enforcement after his significant other, Heather, called "911" when Walker, according to her report, stated that he was going to go out and end his life with a handgun. Heather agreed to go to the emergency department so she could speak to the medical staff and the mental health clinician.

Law enforcement located Walker at his residence where he stated that this was "all a misunderstanding" and he had "never made a statement about killing himself and he was not suicidal." They explained that they take any call related to suicide very seriously and he would need to be brought in for a mental health assessment. Walker cooperated with the officers and upon arrival at the emergency department was cooperative and answered all of the emergency room physician's questions. The doctor did not request lab work as Walker denied the use of alcohol and that his statement regarding not being suicidal was credible.

The physician also spoke to Heather who provided a whole different story. The doctor did not know who to believe but felt it was best that Walker go to the inpatient psych unit for further assessment. The mental health clinician was called in for a risk assessment since Walker was not willing to agree to voluntary admission to the inpatient psychiatric unit. The doctor instructs the clinician that he "needs some help sorting this one out."

Upon arrival at the emergency department and prior to speaking to the medical staff Heather managed to corner the mental health clinician and gave him an ear-full. She states that Walker had been making these types of statements for at least 2 weeks and is even more adamant about ending his life when he is intoxicated. She became more concerned when the frequency of these statements increased after he was terminated 3 days ago from his job as a construction worker. Heather states he has been drinking everyday since being fired from his job. When she would question him about this Walker would shrug it off and state that "lots of people think about suicide but he would never do that to her." Heather tells the clinician that Walker has weapons in their residence and when he does talk about suicide he states that he "will just blow his brains out." During this conversation Heather is crying and states she desperately loves

112

Walker and that she did not know what else to do but to call "911." Now she is fearful that Walker will not want to be with her any longer.

The mental health clinician thanks Heather for the information and enters the emergency department where he observes Walker sitting on the bed carrying on an animated conversation about fishing and camping with the security guard. They had never met but had mutual friends. The clinician introduced himself and Walker stated "it's nice to meet you, Doc." The clinician explained that he was not a doctor and told Walker that he was a mental health risk assessment specialist and that he was here to speak to him about the reason why Walker was in the hospital at this time. Walker stated that he would be glad to visit with him so this "misunderstanding could be cleared up and he could get home."

Armed with the collateral information from Heather, the clinician was able to quickly focus in on the specifics related to the risk assessment. Walker adamantly denied making a suicide statement in the last 24 hours. He did admit to making a statement about "just wishing this part of life were over" but he states he would "never take his life." He does admit that he has weapons in his residence and states that he has not fired his handguns for about 18 months. They are locked in a safe and he has the key at his residence.

Walker states that he has never been treated for mental health issues and tends to minimize his drinking by stating that he drinks 1 or 2 beers on the weekend nights and does not drink at all during the week. He denies that he had drunk any alcohol today but when questioned more he states that he "maybe had a beer today." He still has a deep love for Heather and he does not hold this against her.

At this time the clinician suspends the interview and asks the physician to do some lab work to determine how much alcohol Walker had in his system. The clinician interviews another patient at the emergency department while waiting for the lab results. Once the lab results are back it is found that Walker has a Blood Alcohol Level of 0.090 which is under the recommended limit for mental health risk assessment.

The clinician concludes the risk assessment and consults with the emergency room physician as well as the on-call psychiatrist who both agree that Walker's story does not match Heather's story and this evokes quite a lot of concern.

<u>Treatment History</u>

No previous treatment history.

<u>Disposition</u>

The mental health clinician concluded that Walker is less credible in his reporting than his significant other, Heather. His minimizing of both his suicidal statements and his usage of alcohol are red flags for the clinician who has no choice but to push for admission to the inpatient psychiatric unit.

The clinician decides to enlist Heather's help to get Walker to realize that he needs treatment. After speaking to Heather about the goals and what her expectations could be of Walker, the clinician facilitates a meeting between Heather and Walker. Heather and the clinician both push hard for Walker to just voluntarily go to the inpatient unit. The meeting went poorly and Walker continues to deny suicidal ideation and a suicide plan. Heather leaves the emergency department in tears. Walker states that she is "making a big deal out of nothing."

Having no other option to keep his patient safe, the clinician wrote paperwork for an involuntary admission to the psychiatric unit. He deemed that Walker was an imminent risk to himself due to his suicidal ideation with a specific suicide plan. He needed to be detained for his safety as well as the safety of the community.

Upon serving the paperwork, Walker became angry and verbally aggressive towards the mental health clinician. He threatened to sue the clinician, the physician, the security guard, and the hospital for detaining him against his will. The emergency room physician ordered a combination of Benedryl, Ativan and Haldol and asked for a "show of force" in order to gain his cooperation for the injection. The medical staff administered the injection to ensure Walker's as well as the staff's physical safety. He soon became sleepy and laid down on the bed in his room and soon was snoring away.

He was transported by ambulance to the inpatient psychiatric hospital.

<u>This patient was involuntarily admitted after considering the following information:</u>

- Suicide plan in place with access to means
- Outpatient options cannot adequately ensured his safety

Case Study #9: He Said She Said. (Version Two)

<u>Presenting Problem</u>

Walker, a 36-year-old male, is brought to the emergency department by law enforcement after his significant other, Heather, called "911" when Walker, according to her report, stated that he was going to go out and end his life with a handgun. Heather agreed to go to the emergency department so she could speak to the medical staff and the mental health clinician.

Law enforcement located Walker at his residence where he stated that this was "all a misunderstanding" and he had "never made a statement about killing himself and he was not suicidal." They explained that they take any call related to suicide very seriously and he would need to be brought in for a mental health assessment. Walker cooperated with the officers and upon arrival at the emergency department was cooperative and answered all of the emergency room physician's questions. The doctor did not request lab work as Walker denied the use of alcohol and that his statement regarding not being suicidal was credible.

The physician also spoke to Heather who provided a whole different story. The doctor did not know who to believe but felt it was best that Walker go to the inpatient psych unit for further assessment. The mental health clinician was called in for a risk assessment since Walker was not willing to agree to voluntary admission to the inpatient psychiatric unit. The doctor instructs the clinician that he "needs some help sorting this one out."

Upon arrival at the emergency department and prior to speaking to the medical staff Heather managed to corner the mental health clinician and gave him an ear-full. She states that Walker had been making these types of statements for at least 2 weeks and is even more adamant about ending his life when he is intoxicated. She became more concerned when the frequency of these statements increased after he was terminated 3 days ago from his job as a construction worker. Heather states he has been drinking everyday since being fired from his job. When she would question him about this Walker would shrug it off and state that "lots of people think about suicide but he would never do that to her." Heather tells the clinician that Walker has weapons in their residence and when he does talk about suicide he states that he "will just blow his brains out." During this conversation Heather is crying and states she desperately loves Walker and that she did not know what else to do but to call "911." Now she is fearful that Walker will not want to be with her any longer.

The mental health clinician thanks Heather for the information and enters the emergency department where he observes Walker sitting on the bed carrying on an animated conversation about fishing and camping with the security guard. They had never met but had mutual friends. The clinician introduced himself and Walker stated "it's nice to meet you, Doc." The clinician explained that he was not a doctor and told Walker that he was a mental health risk assessment specialist and that he was here to speak to him about the reason why Walker was in the hospital at this time. Walker stated that he would be glad to visit with him so this "misunderstanding could be cleared up and he could get home."

Armed with the collateral information from Heather, the clinician was able to quickly focus in on the specifics related to the risk assessment. Walker adamantly denied making a suicide statement in the last 24 hours or at any time for that matter. He did admit to making a statement about "just wishing this part of life were over" but he states he would "never take his life." He does admit that he has weapons in his residence and states that he has not fired his handguns for about 18 months. They are locked in a safe and he has the key at his residence.

Walker states that he has never been treated for mental health issues and did admit to drinking 1 or 2 beers on the weekend nights and does not drink at all during the week. He denies that he had drunk any alcohol today. He also states that he was not fired from his job, he has been laid off for 2 weeks while waiting for the next job to start.

Walker tells the clinician that he and Heather have been going through a rough time and he feels himself wanting to pull away from her. He cares for her but is not sure where the relationship is going. Walker states that Heather has been becoming more desperate in trying to maintain their relationship and has been stirring up conflicts so Walker has to continue to address the conflicts rather than address their relationship issues. He then went on to tell the clinician that Heather has alienated most of his friends and now is working her way through his family as well. This is not the "first time she has alleged that I was suicidal" and "frankly, I am tired of it." Walker gave the clinician permission to contact his parents who live in another town. They have been acutely aware of the issues and also have a great relationship with their son.

During the conversation with Walker's mother the facts were confirmed and the clinician thanked her for her time. Walker's mother has never known her son to make a suicidal statement or even be depressed for that matter. She expresses concern regarding this seemingly unhealthy relationship with Heather.

The clinician concludes the risk assessment and consults with the emergency room physician as well as the on-call psychiatrist who both agree that Walker's story is more credible than Heather's story.

Treatment History

No previous treatment history.

Disposition

The mental health clinician concluded that Walker is more credible in his reporting than his significant other, Heather. He adamantly denies suicidal statements and the clinician recommends discharging this patient.

Walker decided to take a break from the chaos of this relationship and spend the weekend at his sister's residence. He decided not to tell Heather where he was going. Walker's sister agreed to come pick him up at the hospital since he was transported here by law enforcement. The clinician also warned Walker about the possible detrimental effects of alcohol use and he clearly understood the implications of this warning. He was encouraged to seek help related to chemical addiction. He will seek an outpatient chemical dependency evaluation.

He decided to deal with the "Heather issue" after he has some time to clear his head. The clinician then met with Heather and told her that Walker was being discharged and did not want to see her at this time. She flew into a rage and stomped out of the hospital waiting room yelling, "It will be on your @ * & # head when he kills himself."

<u>This patient was discharged after considering
the following information:</u>

- Collateral contact with parents confirming his story
- Family support and patient's agreement to stay with sister
- Walker does not meet admission criteria
- Willingness to engage in chemical dependency assessment

Common Psychiatric Medications

This list provides the common medications used in psychiatry to treat mental illness.

Anti-depressants

SSRIs *(Serotonin Reuptake Inhibitors)*

Celexa -	Citalopram
Lexapro -	Escitalopram
Prozac -	Fluoxetine
Luvox -	Fluvoxamine
Paxil -	Paroxetine
Zoloft -	Sertraline

SNRIs *(Serotonin-Norepinephrine Reuptake Inhibitors)*

Cymbalta -	Duloxetine
Effexor -	Venlafaxine
Pristiq -	Desvenlafaxine

Norepinephrine *(dopamine reuptake inhibitor)*

Wellbutrin –	Bupropion

Tricyclic antidepressants

Elavil -	Amitriptyline
Anafranil -	Clomipramine
Sinequan -	Doxepin
Tofranil -	Imipramine

MAOIs: *(MonoAmine Oxidase Inhibitors)*

Marplan -	Isocarboxazid
Aurorix -	Moclobemide
Nardil -	Phenelzine
Eldepryl -	Selegiline
Parnate –	Tranylcypromine

Anti-Anxiety Agents (Anxiolytic)

Benzodiazepines

Xanax -	Alprazolam
Librium -	Chlordiazepoxide
Klonopin -	Clonazepam
Valium -	Diazepam
Etilaam -	Etizolam
Ativan -	Lorazepam
Serax –	Oxazepam

Antipsychotics

Atypical Antipsychotics *(newer)*

Clozaril -	Clozapine
Zyprexa –	Olanzapine
Risperdal –	Risperidone
Seroquel –	Quetiapine
Geodon –	Ziprasidone
Solian –	Amisulpride
Saphris –	Asenapine
Invega –	Paliperidone
Latuda –	Lurasidone

Typical Antipsychotics (older)

Haldol -	Haloperidol
Inapsine -	Droperidol
Thorazine -	Chlorpromazine
Prolixin –	Fluphenazine
Trilafon –	Perphenazine
Compazine -	Prochlorperazine
Mellaril -	Thioridazine
Stelazine -	Trifluoperazine
Navane –	Thiothixene

Mood Stabilizers

Anticonvulsants

Depakote, Depakene -	Valproic acid
Lamictal -	Lamotrigine
Tegretol -	Carbamazepine
Trileptal -	Oxcarbazepine
Neurontin -	Gabapentin
Topamax -	Topiramate
Lithium	

ADHD Medications

Stimulants	Non stimulants
Adderall	Strattera
Dexedrine	Intuniv
Focalin	Tenex
Ritalin	
Concerta	

Definition Of Terms Related To Activity

Abulia	Decreased activity due to lack of ability or power to execute action, despite a desire to do so. Slow in performing simple cognitive tasks, such as counting backward.
Agitation	Emotionally distressed, cannot sit still or attend, gives evidence of heightened tension.
Akethisia	A feeling of motoric restlessness, particularly of the legs (diagnoses by patient's subjective report.)
Akinesia	A marked reduction in accessory motor activity. (arm swinging, blinking, swallowing, posture adjustment, differentiated from paralysis)
Athetoid Movements	Abnormal movements that are slow, writhing, involuntary and involving the extremities (often described as snakelike)
Autonomic Movements	Involuntary movement that occur in the setting of altered consciousness; also called automatisms.
Bradykinesia	A slowing of motor activity
Cataplexy	Temporary state of sudden involuntary muscle relaxation causing loss of postural tone, in the setting of intact consciousness.

Dystonia	An episode of involuntary increased tone in a muscle or a group of muscles, frequently an extrapyramidal side effect of antipsychotic drugs.
Echopraxia	Involuntary repetition and imitation of another person's movements inappropriate to the situation.
Extrapyramidal side effects	Drug induced abnormalities of the extrapyramidal systems, commonly but not necessarily resembling idiopathic Parkinson's disease.
Hyperactivity	Excessive motoric activity which may or may not be associated with mental changes.
Lead pipe rigidity	Markedly increased muscle tone and resistance to passive movement independent of the direction of movement. May indicate brain damage, neuroleptic malignant syndrome, or acute withdrawal from dopaminergic medication in a parkinsonian patient.
Mannerism	Peculiar repetitive body movement or action that appears bizarre to the observer because it is exaggerated or out of context and does not resemble known types of involuntary movements.
Motor preservation	Deficient capacity to shift from one motor activity to another.
Parkinsonian Movements	Involuntary movement due to dysfunction of the basal ganglia, including resting tremor,

cogwheeling, muscular rigidity, masked facies, bradykinesia, festinating gait.

Psychomotor retardation	Slowing of body movement secondary to psychic dysfunction.
Resistance	Unconscious or subconscious opposition to attempts by others to help the patient or bring them to an awareness of information or ideas that are conflictual or uncomfortable.
Splitting	A psychological defense mechanism in which other person and things are viewed in extremes. Black, and white, good or bad, no ability to consider compromise.
Stereotypy	A repetitive, purposeless movement. (automatism, mannerism)
Tic	Abnormal sudden, repetitive stereotyped jerky movements of eyes, vocal organs, face, extremities or trunk.
Tremors	Rapidly alternating movements of the extremities, trunk, head and neck, tongue, or lips which occur when the limb or trunk is at rest.
Vigilance	Sustained attention to external stimuli.
Viscosity	Difficulty breaking conversations, excessive talking. (temporal lobe epilepsy, left sided seizure focus)

Waxy flexibility

Also called catalpsy. The patient's posture is held in a fixed position for a prolonged period of time, even in odd positions.

Definition Of Terms Related To Mood

Affect

The external manifestation of a patient's emotions or feeling state.

Affective lability

A state of increased affective mobility. Abrupt, dramatic, usually unprovoked changes in the type of emotion expressed.

Agitation

Restless, motorically, hyperactive, uncomfortable state.

Alexithymia

Deficient awareness of different mood states, diminished capacity to describe their feelings verbally.

Anxious mood

Uncomfortable, tense, apprehensive and vigilant emotional state.

Apathy

Lack of interest and desire, accompanied by decreased reaction to internal and external stimuli.

Appropriate affect

A normal state where the emotion apparent to the interviewer matches the content of speech and thought.

Bunted affect

A state of diminished emotional intensity compared to the content of the conversation. (differentiated from flattened affect)

Depressed mood

An emotional state consistent with sadness and dysphoria.

Dysphoria	An unpleasant and negative mood that is perceived as being uncomfortable.
Euphoria	Elevated, exceedingly happy mood.
Euthymia	A normal mood including the ups and downs of life.
Fixed affect	The unvarying display of one particular affect or emotion throughout the interview.
Flat affect	A state in which there is no emotional expression.
Inappropriate affect	The emotion displayed does not match the speech, thought or context accompanying it. (incongruent affect)
Intensity of affect	The strength of emotional expression.
La belle indifference	Lack of the normally expected concern for an apparently serious condition. This associated with conversion disorder and various neuralgic disorders. Demonstrates a significant lack of insight.
Mobility of affect	The ease and speed with which one moves from the expression of one type of feeling to another.
Mood	A person's predominant emotional or feeling state.

Continued on next page

Range of affect	The variety of emotional expression that an individual communicates during an extended interaction.
Reactivity of affect	The extent to which affect changes in direct response to environmental stimuli.
Restricted affect	A limited or decreased rage of affect.

Source for Definition of Terms:

Paula T. Trzepacz and Robert W. Baker: The Psychiatric Mental Status Examination. New York: Oxford University Press, 1993

Frequently Used Terms And Contacts

_____

_____

_____

_____

_____

_____

_____

_____

_____

_____

_____

_____

_____

Reference Section

Abuse

Canadian Journal of Psychiatry. 1998 Oct; 43(8): 793-800
Childhood sexual and physical abuse and adult self-harm and suicidal behavior: a literature review

International Journal of Adolescent Medical Health. 2007 Jan-Mar; 19(1):45-51
Childhood abuse and adolescent suicidality: a direct link and an indirect link through alcohol and substance misuse

Journal of Adolescent Health. 1992 Mar; 13(2): 128-32
Physical and sexual abuse as predictors of substance use and suicide among pregnant teenagers

Quarterly Journal of Medicine . 2007 May; 100(5): 305-9
Childhood abuse, adult alcohol use disorders and suicidal behavior

Alcohol

Alcohol and Alcoholism. 2006 Sep-Oct; 41(5): 473-8
The association between alcohol misuse and suicidal behaviour

Alcoholism: Clinical and Experimental Research. 2004 May; 28(5 Suppl): 18S-28S
Acute alcohol use and suicidal behavior: a review of the literature

Alcoholism: Clinical and Experimental Research. 2004 May; 28(5 Suppl): 77S-88S
Adolescent substance use and suicidal behavior: a review with implications for treatment.

Experimental Research. 2006 Jun; 30(6): 998-1005
Suicide attempts among substance use disorder patients: an initial step toward a decision tree for suicide management.

Clinical Psychology Review. 2001 Jul; 21(5): 797-811
Alcohol and suicidal behavior

Journal of Depression and Anxiety. 2001; 14(3) :186-91
Adolescent substance abuse and suicide

Drug and Alcohol Dependence. 2004 Dec 7; 76 Suppl: S11-9
Association of alcohol and drug use disorders and completed suicide: an empirical review of cohort studies.

International Journal of Adolescent Medicine and Health . 2005 Jul-Sep;
17(3): 197-203
Alcohol and adolescent suicide

International Journal of Adolescent Medicine and Health . 2007 Jan-Mar;
19(1): 27-35
Suicidality, depression, and alcohol use among adolescents: a review of
empirical findings

International Journal of Circumpolar Health. 2007; 66 Suppl 1: 54-60
Fetal alcohol spectrum disorders and suicidality in a healthcare setting

Journal of Clinical Psychiatry. 1999; 60 Suppl 2: 63-9
Suicide attempts in major affective disorder patients with comorbid
substance use disorders

Journal of Clinical Psychiatry. 1999; 60 Suppl 2: 63-9; discussion 75-6, 113-6
Suicide attempts in major affective disorder patients with comorbid
substance use disorders.

Quarterly Journal of Medicine . 2006 Jan; 99(1): 57-61
Alcohol consumption and suicide

Romanian Journal of Gastroenterology . 2002 Sep; 11(3): 197-204
Effect of ethanol and alcoholic beverages on the gastrointestinal tract in
humans

Scientific World Journal. 2006 Jun 21; 6: 700-6
Alcohol and suicide: neurobiological and clinical aspects

Scientific World Journal. 2006 Oct 31; 6: 1405-11
Risk and protective factors for suicide in patients with alcoholism

Anxiety Disorders

Archives of General Psychiatry. 2005 Nov; 62(11): 1249-57
Anxiety disorders and risk for suicidal ideation and suicide attempts: a
population-based longitudinal study of adults

Current Opinion in Psychiatry. 2008 Jan; 21(1): 51-64
Review Anxiety disorders and suicidal behavior: an update.

Comprehensive Psychiatry. 2001 Nov-Dec; 42(6): 477-81
Alexithymia and suicidality in panic disorder

Journal of Depression and Anxiety. 2006; 23(3): 124-32
Panic and suicidal ideation and suicide attempts: results from the
National Comorbidity Survey

Anxiety Disorders (cont.)

Journal of Abnormal Psychology. 2004 Nov; 113(4): 582-91
Panic disorder and suicide attempt in the National Comorbidity Survey

Journal of Affective Disorders. 2007 Dec; 104(1-3): 203-9
Panic disorder and suicidality: is comorbidity with depression the key?

Journal of Depression and Anxiety. 2008; 25(6): 477-81
Anxiety disorders and risk for suicide attempts: findings from the
Baltimore Epidemiologic Catchment area follow-up study

Journal of Affective Disorders. 2002 Apr; 68(2-3): 183-90
Suicide risk in patients with anxiety disorders: a meta-analysis of the
FDA database

Psychological Medicine. 2007 Mar; 37(3): 431-40
Anxiety disorders and suicidal behaviors in adolescence and young
adulthood: findings from a longitudinal study.

Annals of General Psychiatry. 2007 Sep 5; 6: 23
Prediction and prevention of suicide in patients with unipolar
depression and anxiety

Assessment

CNS Spectrums. 2006 Jun; 11(6): 442-5
The standard of care in suicide risk assessment: An elusive concept.

Nursing Times. 2006 Jan 10-16; 102(2): 36-8
How to use non-verbal signs in assessments of suicide risk

Psychiatry Research. 2001 Dec 31; 105(3): 255-64
Inpatient diagnostic assessments: 1. Accuracy of structured vs.
unstructured interviews

Bipolar Illness

Bipolar Disorder Journal. 2002; 4 Suppl 1: 21-5
Bipolar Disorder Journalers and suicidal behaviour

Bipolar Disorder Journal. 2005 Oct; 7(5): 441-8
Rapid mood switching and suicidality in familial Bipolar Disorder
Journaler

Bipolar Disorder Journal. 2006 Oct; 8(5 Pt 2): 576-85
Prospective study of risk factors for attempted suicide among patients
with Bipolar Disorder Journaler.

Journal of Clinical Psychiatry. 2000; 61 Suppl 9: 47-51
Suicide and Bipolar Disorder Journaler

Journal of Clinical Psychiatry. 2005 Jun; 66(6): 693-704
Suicide and attempted suicide in Bipolar Disorder Journaler: a systematic review of risk factors

Journal of Clinical Psychiatry. 2005 Nov; 66(11): 1456-62
Suicidal ideation and attempts in bipolar I and II disorders.

Journal of Clinical Psychiatry. 2004; 65 Suppl 10: 5-10
Correlates of suicidal behavior and lithium treatment in Bipolar Disorder Journaler

Dissociative Disorders

The Journal of Nervous and Mental Disease. 2008 Jan; 196(1): 29-36
Dissociative disorders and suicidality in psychiatric outpatients

Drugs of Abuse

Addictive Behaviors. 2007 Jul; 32(7): 1395-404
Suicide attempts among individuals with opiate dependence: the critical role of belonging

Addictive Behaviors. 2008 Jan; 33(1): 152-5
Cannabis use and suicidal behaviours in high-school students

Addiction. 2002 Nov; 97(11): 1383-94
Suicide among heroin users: rates, risk factors and methods

Addiction. 2007 Dec; 102(12): 1933-41
Suicidal behaviour and associated risk factors among opioid-dependent individuals: a case-control study

American Journal on Addictions. 2008 Jan-Feb; 17(1): 24-7
Risk factors for suicide attempts in methamphetamine-dependent patients

Archives of General Psychiatry. 2004 Oct; 61(10): 1026-32
Major depressive disorder, suicidal ideation, and suicide attempt in twins discordant for cannabis dependence and early-onset cannabis use

Drug and Alcohol Dependence. 2003 May 1;70(1):101-4
Cocaine use disorders and suicidal ideation

Drug and Alcohol Review. 2003 Mar; 22(1): 21-5
The relationship of conduct disorder to attempted suicide and drug use history among methadone maintenance patients

Drugs of Abuse (cont.)

Drug and Alcohol Review. 2008 May; 27(3): 253-62
Major physical and psychological harms of methamphetamine use

The Journal of Nervous and Mental Disease. 2005 Jul; 193(7): 431-7
Predictors of high rates of suicidal ideation among drug users

Medical Journal of Australia. 1994 Jun 6;160(11): 731
Cannabis and suicide

Suicide and Life-Threatening Behavior. 2007 Aug; 37(4): 475-81
Heroin addicts reporting previous heroin overdoses also report suicide attempts

Eating Disorders and Related Topics

Clinical Psychology Review. 2006 Oct; 26(6): 769-82
Review Suicidality in eating disorders: occurrence, correlates, and clinical implications.

Clinical Psychology Review. 2006 Oct; 26(6): 769-82
Suicidality in eating disorders: occurrence, correlates, and clinical implications

Journal of Clinical Psychiatry. 2005 Jun; 66(6): 717-25
Suicidal ideation and suicide attempts in body dysmorphic disorder.

Pediactrics International. 2006 Aug; 48(4): 374-81
Suicide attempts versus suicidal ideation in bulimic female adolescents

Psychosomatic Medicine. 2008 Apr; 70(3): 378-83
Suicide attempts in anorexia nervosa

Scientific World Journal. 2005 Sep 28; 5: 803-11
A review of eating disorders and suicide risk in adolescence.

Legal Issues

Behavioral Sciences and the Law . 2004; 22(5): 697-713
Legal issues of professional negligence in suicide cases

Journal of Psychosocial Nursing and Mental Health Services. 2006 Dec; 44(12): 8
Suicide and documentation: a must-read

Journal of Psychosocial Nursing and Mental Health Services. 2006 Jul; 44(7): 18-24
Suicide and documentation: don't let the pen kill your career.

Medical Issues

Acta Psychiatrica Scandinavia 2003 Jan; 107(1): 41-4
   Characteristics of HIV patients who attempt suicide

Alimentary Pharmacology Therapeutics. 2007 Jul 15; 26(2): 183-93
   Systematic review: the prevalence of suicidal behaviour in patients with
   chronic abdominal pain and irritable bowel syndrome.

British Journal of Psychiatry. 2006 Feb; 188: 192
   Akathisia as a risk factor for suicide.

Brain Injury. 2007 Dec; 21(13-14): 1335-51
   Suicidality in people surviving a traumatic Brain Injury: prevalence, risk
   factors and implications for clinical management.

Clinical Journal of Pain. 2008 Mar-Apr; 24(3): 204-10
   Chronic pain conditions and suicidal ideation and suicide attempts: an
   epidemiologic perspective

Current Treatment Options in Neurology. 2008 Sep; 10(5): 363-76
   Allergy: a risk factor for suicide?

Epilepsy & Behavior. 2003 Oct; 4 Suppl 3: S31-8
   Rates and risk factors for suicide, suicidal ideation, and suicide attempts
   in chronic epilepsy

Harvard Review of Psychiatry. 1993 May-Jun; 1(1): 27-35
   Suicide risk in patients with human immunodeficiency virus infection
   and acquired immunodeficiency syndrome

Journal of Hospital Medicine. 2000 May; 61(5): 311-4
   HIV, childbirth and suicidal behaviour: a review

Journal of Clinical Oncology. 2008 Aug 11
   Cancer and the Risk of Suicide in Older Americans

Journal of Nervous and Mental Disease. 1992 May; 180(5): 339
   Reported association of akathisia with suicide

Medical Issues (cont).

Journal of the American Medical Association. 2000 Dec 13; 284(22): 2907-11
Depression, hopelessness, and desire for hastened death in terminally ill patients with cancer

Journal of Palliative Medicine. 2006 Oct; 20(7): 693-701
Desire for hastened death in patients with advanced disease and the evidence base of clinical guidelines: a systematic review

Psychological Medicine. 2006 Jul; 36(7): 901-12
Suicidal behaviour and the menstrual cycle

Psychological Medicine. 2006 May; 36(5): 575-86
Suicidality in chronic pain: a review of the prevalence, risk factors and psychological links.

Tumori: A Journal of Experimental and Clinical Oncology. 2002 May-Jun; 88(3): 193-9
Suicide and suicidal thoughts in cancer patients

===

Medication

Journal of the American Psychiatric Association. 2006 May; 163(5): 813-21
The risk of suicide with selective serotonin reuptake inhibitors in the elderly

Journal of the American Psychiatric Association. 2007 Dec; 164(12): 1907-8
SSRI prescriptions and the rate of suicide

Annals of Epidemiology. 1997 Nov; 7(8): 568-74
Risk of suicide attempts after benzodiazepine and/or antidepressant use.

Archives of General Psychiatry. 2005 Feb; 62(2): 165-72
The relationship between antidepressant medication use and rate of suicide

Australian and New Zealand Journal of Psychiatry. 2006 Nov-Dec; 40 (11-12): 941-50
How have the selective serotonin reuptake inhibitor antidepressants affected suicide mortality

British Medical Journal. 2005 Feb 19; 330(7488): 396
Association between suicide attempts and selective serotonin reuptake inhibitors: systematic review of randomised controlled trials.

Current Drug Safety Journalety. 2006 Jan; 1(1): 59-62
SSRIs, suicide and violent behavior: is there a need for a better definition of the depressive state

Drug Safety Journal. 2007; 30(2): 123-42
  Suicidality and antiepileptic drugs: is there a link?

Encephale. 1996 Dec; 22 Spec No 4: 40-5
  Suicide and psychotropic drugs

Journal of Clinical Psychiatry. 2004 Nov; 65(11): 1456-62
  Antidepressants and suicide risk in the United States, 1985-1999

Journal of Psychosocial Nursing and Mental Health Services. 2007 Jul; 45(7): 15-9
  Antidepressants & suicide: putting the risk in perspective

Journal of the American Medical Association. 2004 Jul 21; 292(3): 338-43
  Antidepressants and the risk of suicidal behaviors

Progress in Brain Research Journal. 2008; 172: 307-15
  The role of dopamine and serotonin in suicidal behaviour and aggression

Mood Disorders

Acta Psychiatrica Scandinavia 2006 Sep; 114(3): 151-8
  Prospective studies of suicidal behavior in major depressive and Bipolar Disorder Journalers: what is the evidence for predictive risk factors?

Journal of the American Psychiatric Association. 2000 Dec; 157(12): 1925-32
  Affective disorders and suicide risk: a reexamination.

Journal of the American Psychiatric Association. 2007 Jan; 164(1): 134-41
  Sex differences in clinical predictors of suicidal acts after major depression: a prospective study

Comprehensive Psychiatry. 2006 Sep-Oct; 47(5): 334-41
  Lifetime rhythmicity and mania as correlates of suicidal ideation and attempts in mood disorders

Current Opinion in Psychiatry. 2007 Jan; 20(1): 17-22
  Suicide risk in mood disorders

Journal of Depression and Anxiety. 2001; 14(3): 177-82
  Suicide in mood disorders (adolescents & children)

Journal of Affective Disorders. 2008 Oct 7
  Do major depressive disorder and dysthymic disorder confer differential risk for suicide?

Mood disorders (cont.)

Journal of Clinical Psychiatry. 2001; 62 Suppl 25: 27-30
  Mood disorders and suicide.

Journal of Clinical Psychiatry. 2002 Oct; 63(10): 866-73
  A longitudinal view of triggers and thresholds of suicidal behavior in depression

Minerva Pediatrica. 2008 Apr; 60(2): 201-9
  Depression and suicidal behavior in alcohol abusing adolescents: possible role of selenium deficiency

Progress in Neuro-Psychopharmacology and Biological Psychiatry. 2006 Jul; 30(5): 815-26
  Darwinian models of depression: a review of evolutionary accounts of mood and mood disorders.

Obsessive-Compulsive Personality Disorder

Journal of Clinical Psychiatry. 2007 Nov; 68(11): 1741-50
  Suicidal behavior in obsessive-compulsive disorder

Psychopathology. 2007; 40(3): 184-90
  The impact of obsessive-compulsive personality disorder on the suicidal risk of patients with mood disorders

Personality Disorder

American Journal of Geriatric Psychiatry. 2007 Sep; 15(9): 734-41
  Narcissistic personality and vulnerability to late-life suicidality

Journal of the American Psychiatric Association. 2006 Jan; 163(1): 20-6
  Borderline personality disorder and suicidality

Canadian Journal of Psychiatry. 2003 Jun; 48(5): 301-10
  Assessing suicidal youth with antisocial, borderline, or narcissistic personality disorder

Journal of Clinical Psychiatry. 2007 May; 68(5): 721-9
  Risk factors for suicide completion in borderline personality disorder: a case-control study of cluster B comorbidity and impulsive aggression.

Journal of Personality Disorders. 2004 Jun; 18(3): 226-39
  Suicidal behavior in borderline personality disorder: prevalence, risk factors, prediction, and prevention

Psychiatric Services. 2002 Jun; 53(6): 738-42
  Chronic suicidality among patients with borderline personality disorder

Posttraumatic Stress Disorder

Journal of Psychiatric Practice. 2008 Jul; 14(4): 195
  PTSD and Suicide

Psychosomatic Medicine. 2007 Apr; 69(3): 242-8
  Physical and mental comorbidity, disability, and suicidal behavior
  associated with posttraumatic stress disorder in a large community
  sample

Schizophrenia Research Journal. 2006 May; 84(1): 165-9
  Comorbid posttraumatic stress disorder is associated with suicidality in
  male veterans with schizophrenia or schizoaffective disorder

---

Schizophrenia

Journal of Psychopharmacology Journal of Psychopharmacology. 2001 Jun;
15(2): 127-35
  Suicide and schizophrenia

Archives of General Psychiatry. 2005 Mar; 62(3): 247-53
  The lifetime risk of suicide in schizophrenia: a reexamination

Current Psychiatry Reports. 2002 Aug; 4(4): 279-83
  Suicidality in schizophrenia: a review of the evidence for risk factors
  and treatment options.

Journal of Clinical Psychiatry. 2005 May; 66(5): 579-85
  Risk factors for completed suicide in schizophrenia

Psychology and Psychotherapy. 2008 Mar; 81(Pt 1): 55-77
  Suicide risk in schizophrenia: explanatory models and clinical
  implications, The Schematic Appraisal Model of Suicide (SAMS).

Suicide

Annals of Clinical Psychiatry. 2001 Jun; 13(2): 93-101
Sleep and suicide in psychiatric patients

Annual Review of Clinical Psychology. 2006; 2: 237-66
Attempted and completed suicide in adolescence

Archives of Internal Medicine. 1996 Mar 11; 156(5): 521-5
A prospective study of coffee drinking and suicide in women

Canadian Journal of Psychiatry. 2003 Jun; 48(5): 292-300
The neurobiology of suicide and suicidality

Crisis. 2001; 22(3): 125-31
Suicidal behavior in patients with adjustment disorders

Crisis. 2004; 25(4): 147-55
Psychiatric diagnoses and suicide: revisiting the evidence

Current Opinion in Psychiatry. 2006 May; 19(3): 288-93
Sleep and youth suicidal behavior: a neglected field

Death Studies. 2006 Apr; 30(3): 269-79
Recognition of suicide risk according to the characteristics of the
suicide process

Drugs & Aging. 2002; 19(1): 11-24
Identification of suicidal ideation and prevention of suicidal behaviour
in the elderly

European Journal of Epidemiology. 2000; 16(9): 789-91
Heavy coffee drinking and the risk of suicide

Harvard Review of Psychiatry. 2004 Jan-Feb; 12(1): 1-13
Genetics of suicide: an overview

Journal of Abnormal Psychology. 2006 Nov; 115(4): 842-9
Predictors of suicide attempts: state and trait components.

Military Medicine. 2005 Jul; 170(7): 580-4
Suicide in the Army: a review of current information

Pediatrics. 2001 Aug; 108(2): E30
Adoption as a risk factor for attempted suicide during adolescence

Psychiatry Research. 1991 Mar; 36(3): 265-77
Sleep, depression, and suicide

Psychological Medicine. 2003 Apr; 33(3): 395-405
Psychological autopsy studies of suicide: a systematic review

Suicide and Life-Threatening Behavior. 2000 Summer; 30(2): 145-62
Suicide: a 15-year review of the sociological literature. Part I: cultural and economic factors

Suicide and Life-Threatening Behavior. 2000 Summer; 30(2): 163-76
Suicide: a 15-year review of the sociological literature. Part II: modernization and social integration perspectives

Suicide and Life-Threatening Behavior. 2004 Winter; 34(4): 386-94
Desperation and other affective states in suicidal patients

Violence / Impulsivity

Current Psychiatry Reports. 2007 Dec; 9(6): 460-6
The relationship of impulsive aggressiveness to suicidality and other depression-linked behaviors.

The Journal of Nervous and Mental Disease. 2001 Mar; 189(3): 162-7
Anger, impulsivity, social support, and suicide risk in patients with posttraumatic stress disorder

Pharmacopsychiatry. 1995 Oct; 28 Suppl 2: 47-57
Outward and inward directed aggressiveness: the interaction between violence and suicidality

Psychiatric Clinics of North America. 2000 Mar; 23(1): 11-25
The biology of impulsivity and suicidality

Psychological Medicine. 2006 Dec; 36(12): 1779-88
Aggressiveness, not impulsiveness or hostility, distinguishes suicide attempters with major depression

Notes

Psychrisk also provides training and consultation for mental health centers, emergency department and law enforcement agencies.

For more information visit
www.psychrisk.com